Clinical Ophthalmology

D0351423

To my family
J. A. B., A. G. K. B. and M. J. K. B.

James Bankes sadly died on 16 October 1993 aged 58 years at home after a long and painful battle with cancer which he fought with outstanding courage and dignity.

He finished the text of the third edition shortly before his death.

For Churchill Livingstone

Publisher: Michael Parkinson
Project Editor: Dilys Jones
Copy Editor: Kathryn Whyman
Design: Design Resources Unit
Production Controllers: Debra Barrie, Nancy Arnott
Sales Promotion Executive: Duncan Jones

Clinical Ophthalmology

A TEXT AND COLOUR ATLAS

James L. Kennerley Bankes MB BS (Lond), FRCS (Eng), FRCOphth
Formerly Consultant Ophthalmic Surgeon St Mary's Hospital and Western Ophthalmic Hospital, London
Hon. Senior Clinical Lecturer St Mary's Hospital Medical School (University of London)
Hon. Consultant Ophthalmic Surgeon The Royal Hospital, Chelsea, London

THIRD EDITION

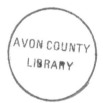

CHURCHILL LIVINGSTONE
EDINBURGH LONDON MADRID MELBOURNE NEW YORK AND TOKYO 1994

CHURCHILL LIVINGSTONE
Medical Division of Longman Group UK Limited

Distributed in the United States of America by Churchill
Livingstone Inc., 650 Avenue of the Americas, New York,
N.Y. 10011, and by associated companies, branches and
representatives throughout the world.

First edition 1982
Second edition 1987
Third edition 1994

ISBN 0 443 04819 3

British Library Cataloguing in Publication Data
A catalogue record for this book is available from the British Library.

Library of Congress Cataloging in Publication Data
A catalog record for this book is available from the Library of Congress.

The
publisher's
policy is to use
**paper manufactured
from sustainable forests**

Printed in Hong Kong
LYP/01

Contents

Preface to the Third Edition

Although the principles of ophthalmology remain unaltered, there have been new techniques in treatment, particularly in surgery, which have been developed. Especially, the now routine use of intraocular lens implants and refractive surgery are mentioned, although the finer details of surgical technique are not appropriate for this book.

Observation remains the key to success in diagnosis and treatment in ophthalmology and the budding ophthalmologist and student is indeed fortunate in having at his or her fingertips precise equipment for this purpose.

London, 1993   J. L. K. B.

Preface to the First Edition

This book is written for those requiring some specialised knowledge of ophthalmology in their work and it is hoped that the needs of medical students, general medical practitioners and those beginning a career in ophthalmology will be met. Optometry students and optometrists have a need for a basic book in ophthalmology and it is hoped that this book will fulfil their requirements. There is much sophistication of instrumentation and surgery in ophthalmology which often obscures the fundamental unchanging facts and principles of the subject. All that is not essential for the non-specialist has been omitted, but conversely it is hoped that the vital fundamental information for clinical practice and reference is contained in this book. The book contains many colour illustrations, together with a few diagrams which assume a basic knowledge of anatomy and physiology. One chapter on rapid changes in refractive errors has the optometry student and optometrist much in mind, but may also prove of interest to the medical practitioner. Where appropriate, detailed treatments are given because the general medical practitioner often has to give the primary ophthalmological treatment.

London, 1982   J. L. K. B.

Acknowledgements

My colleagues at St Mary's Hospital and the Western Ophthalmic Hospital have as always given me great assistance and co-operation, particularly R. J. Marsh, C. Townsend and E. Schulenburg. Miss Susan Ford has given considerable help and skill in many of the illustrations and I am indebted to her in this essential work.

Miss Cyrilla Chatfield has performed all the preparation of the typescript and organisation of this third edition. I wish to thank her especially for this vital part in the production of the book.

My family have urged me on with this third edition when spirits were flagging and I owe them my continuing gratitude. It is particularly pleasing that they can now provide help in the medical content of the book as well.

1

Examination of the eye: use of instruments

A careful history from the patient together with accurate observation of the eyes and their surroundings will usually lead to a clear diagnosis without any special investigations. Constant observation of the normal will easily lead to the rapid identification of the abnormal. Bear in mind the simple anatomy of the eye (Fig. 1.1, 1.2).

It should be remembered that patients with any eye condition are abnormally anxious. However trivial the complaint may be to the clinician the majority of patients have one major fear; the fear of blindness.

THE HISTORY

A complete and accurate history of the patient's complaint is essential. The particular character of the ocular and visual symptoms and their site, duration and frequency brings home the old medical adage of the patient telling the clinician the diagnosis if the clinician will listen and accurately interpret the symptoms.

Details of *past ophthalmic, medical* and *family history* will all aid diagnosis. In infants and children additional *birth and neonatal history* will also give further evidence.

THE EXAMINATION

Estimation of visual acuity

The standard, internally illuminated Snellen Chart consists of rows of letters diminishing in size from the top of the chart downwards. Each row of letters is designated by a ratio of the test distance (6 m or 20 ft) to the distance a normal person could read that sized letter. Hence the top letter on the chart is designated 6/60 because a normal person could read that large letter at 60 m. The lowest line of letters on the chart is designated 6/6 (20/20 in North America) which is the standard normal vision and the size of letter seen by a normal person at 6 m.

The patient is seated 6 m from the test chart and each eye is covered in turn. Any distance spectacles should be worn for this

1

Fig. 1.1
Horizontal section of eye.
(Reproduced with kind permission of
the Hoya Corporation, Japan)

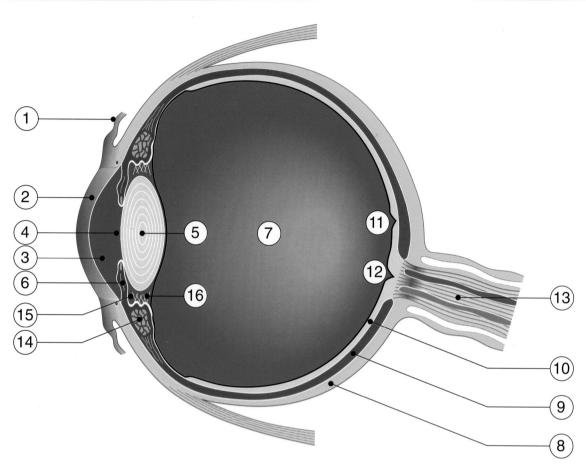

Horizontal section of the eye

1	Conjunctiva	9	Choroid
2	Cornea	10	Retina
3	Anterior chamber	11	Fovea (centralis)
4	Pupil	12	Optic disk
5	Lens	13	Optic nerve
6	Iris	14	Ciliary body
7	Vitreous body	15	Posterior chamber
8	Sclera	16	Zinn's zonule

Fig. 1.2
Vertical section of eye. (Reproduced with kind permission of the Hoya Corporation, Japan)

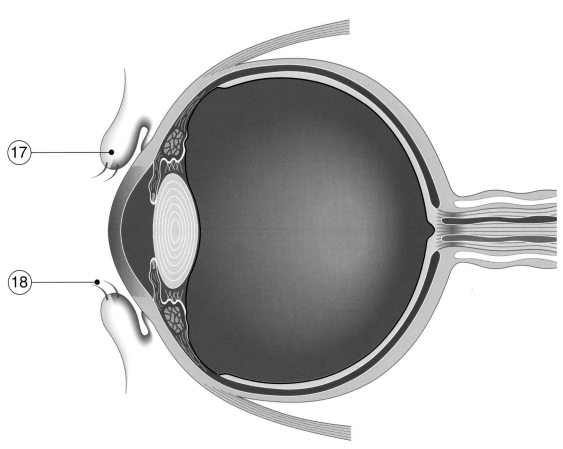

Vertical section of the eye

17 Eyelid
18 Eyelashes

Fig. 1.3
The Snellen chart

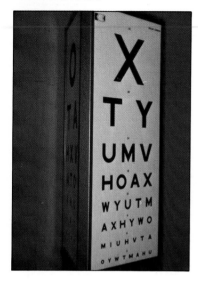

essentially distance test. Should the patient's visual acuity be so poor that even the top letter on the chart cannot be seen then he is brought to 3 m (10 ft) from the chart. If the top letter is then seen the visual acuity would be 3/60 but if not then the examiner holds up his hand at 1m and asks the patient: 'How many fingers am I holding up?' A correct reply will give a designated vision of counting fingers (CF) at 1 m (or less). Failing accurate finger counting the hand is moved in front of the eye and the patient is asked if any movement can be detected. This is designated hand movements (HM). Failure to see the examiner's hand moving means vision is slight only and this is designated perception of light (PL), or absent perception of light, according to whether a bright light can be detected when shone on the eye (Fig. 1.3).

For illiterate patients, and those unfamiliar with the Roman alphabet, letter E's of the standard test sizes and facing different directions may be used, the patient indicating with his own hand the direction of the legs of the E.

For children from age 3 years and over the Sheridan-Gardiner test is excellent. The examiner holds at a 6 m distance a card on which is a single test letter and the child is asked to point to the matching letter on his own card. He thus does not name the letter but merely matches it with his own card (Fig. 1.4).

Pin-hole test
Looking through a tiny hole in a card held close to the eye is useful when testing visual acuity where a high refractive error is present and the patient's spectacles are not available. The hole in the card (easily made by a pin pushed through a card about 50 mm in diameter) allows only central light rays into the eye and eliminates the blurring of vision due to the refractive error. In general an improved visual acuity through the pin-hole indicates a refractive error, rather than a pathological condition, is the likely cause of the reduced visual acuity.

Fig. 1.4
The Sheridan-Gardiner test

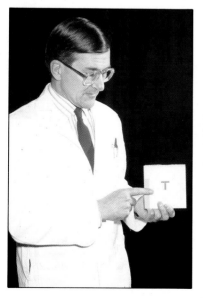

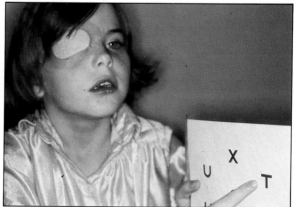

Visual fields

An accurate estimation of the field of vision can be obtained very simply. The patient and examiner are seated facing each other at the same level. With one eye covered by the palm of his hand the patient is asked to fix his gaze on the examiner's nose (a suitable fixation point). The examiner similarly covers his opposite eye and from the periphery of the visual field, each direction in turn, brings in a bright test-object which is a small white or red ball on a long pin (a hat pin). This is the confrontation test.

This test can be surprisingly accurate with practice and is especially useful for a rapid field of vision screening when a central scotoma or hemianopia is suspected (Fig. 1.5).

Fig. 1.5
The confrontation field test

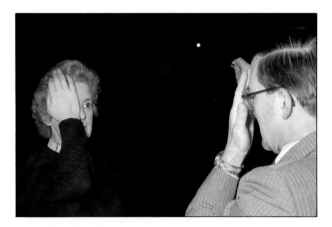

Accurate visual field plotting by various static and kinetic perimetry machines is available to the specialist.

Inspection of face and eyelids

In a good light careful inspection of the face and eyelids will reveal any abnormalities. Details of facial anomalies and especially asymmetry should be noted. The movement of the eyelids should be noted when ocular motility is examined.

Ocular motility

The movements of the eyes are examined in the six cardinal positions of gaze (Fig. 1.6). The patient is asked to follow a fixation

Fig. 1.6
The six cardinal positions of gaze

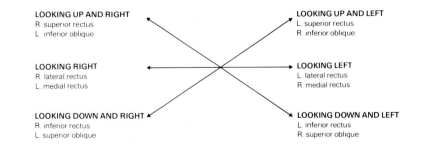

LOOKING UP AND RIGHT
R. superior rectus
L. inferior oblique

LOOKING UP AND LEFT
L. superior rectus
R. inferior oblique

LOOKING RIGHT
R. lateral rectus
L. medial rectus

LOOKING LEFT
L. lateral rectus
R. medial rectus

LOOKING DOWN AND RIGHT
R. inferior rectus
L. superior oblique

LOOKING DOWN AND LEFT
L. inferior rectus
R. superior oblique

target or pen torch light horizontally to right and left and then up and right, down and right, up and left and finally down and left. Any limitation of movement will be revealed indicating the particular weakened muscle (Fig. 1.7).

Fig. 1.7
Extrinsic (extraocular) muscles of eye. (Reproduced with kind permission of the Hoya Corporation, Japan)

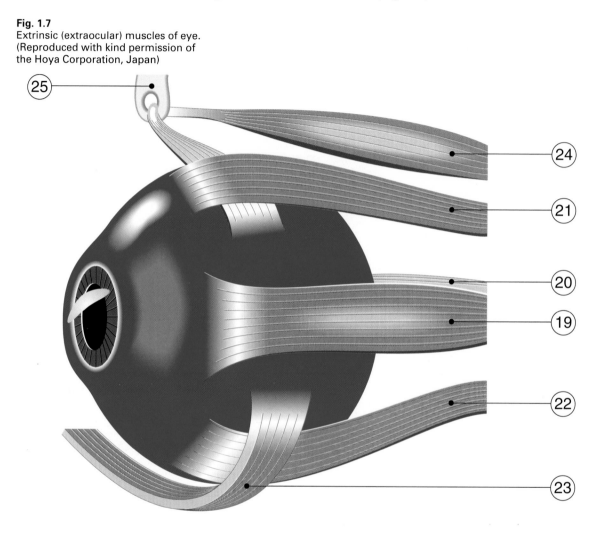

Extrinsic muscles of the eye

19 Lateral rectus
20 Medial rectus
21 Superior rectus
22 Inferior rectus
23 Inferior oblique
24 Superior oblique
25 Trochlea

The pupils

The pupils are normally round and equal in size. Any size or shape anomaly should be noted and the direct light, consensual light and convergence pupil reflexes tested. In eliciting the light pupil reflexes the light should be shone on the central retina (macula) and not obliquely. The convergence reflex is best determined by asking the patient to look at a particular point across the room and then asking him to look at a near object rapidly.

The eye

Inspection of the cornea, conjunctiva, iris, lens and anterior chamber should be made in a good light—daylight is the best. Further detail of the anterior part of the eye can be seen with a simple magnifier (a loupe). The magnifier, say mag. ×6, is held close to the eye and a focusing pen torch is held with the other hand and shone on to the eye from the opposite side. This technique is important in searching for a corneal foreign body, corneal ulceration and flare or a hyphaema in the anterior chamber (Fig. 1.8).

The specialist uses the same focused light and magnifier in the form of the slit lamp microscope (Fig. 1.9).

Fig. 1.8
Examining the outer eye with a simple magnifier

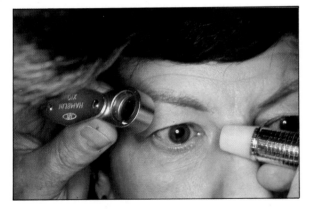

Fig. 1.9
The slit lamp microscope

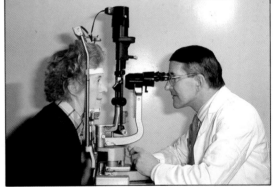

The ophthalmoscope

This instrument allows a view of the interior of the eye; especially the fundus. With the conventional direct ophthalmoscope one eye only is used for observation which therefore does not allow a three dimensional view. The binocular indirect ophthalmoscope allows a stereoscopic or three dimensional view of the interior of the eye and is used by the specialist.

With the direct ophthalmoscope a magnified image is seen. Ideally ophthalmoscopy should be carried out in a darkened room with the patient and examiner seated facing each other at the same level.

The examiner's hand should be placed gently on the patient's forehead with the thumb over the patient's brow and upper eyelid.

Fig. 1.10
Using the direct ophthalmoscope

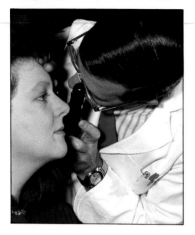

To examine the patient's right eye the examiner uses his own right eye and places his left hand on the patient's forehead, reversed for the left eye examination. The examiner's thumb over the brow and upper eyelid allows the eyelid to be elevated to avoid the eyelashes obstructing the view (Fig. 1.10).

With the patient fixing his gaze on a point across the room the ophthalmoscope light is shone into his pupil and a red fundus reflection (or reflex) will be observed. With a +5 or +6 lens in the ophthalmoscope rack (black numbers) held at about 120 mm from the eye, any opacities in the cornea, lens and vitreous will be visible as silhouettes against the red fundus reflex. This is particularly useful in detecting cataract. The ophthalmoscope is then brought slowly closer to the patient's eye (15 mm is satisfactory) and the ophthalmoscope lens racked to approximately zero until details of the fundus come into view.

Adjustments to the rack of lenses on the ophthalmoscope will be required to obtain a clear fundus picture depending on the refractive error of the patient and the examiner. The optic disc should first be inspected, then the macula, the retinal vessels and finally each quadrant of the fundus in turn.

Ophthalmoscopy requires constant practice. Difficulties in visualising the fundus may occur when:
1. The ophthalmoscope light is poor (poorly charged batteries)
2. The pupil is too small
3. There is too much light scatter from the corneal surface
4. The room is inadequately darkened
5. High myopia is present; in myopia there is a greater magnification of the fundus picture leading to difficulties in orientation and this can be overcome by performing ophthalmoscopy with the patient wearing his distance spectacles
6. Opacities in the media, especially cataract, obscure a good fundus view

Pupil dilation for fundus examination is best achieved using cyclopentolate 1% (Mydrilate) or tropicamide 1% (Mydriacyl) eye drops. After fundus examination reversal of the pupil dilation may be achieved with Pilocarpine 2% drops.

2

Refractive errors

The ideal eye perfectly refracts light entering it to form a precise image on the retina. This refraction depends on the curvature of the cornea and the axial length of the eye (about 24 mm). The perfect refraction of the eye seen in most of the population is called emmetropia.

When the corneal curvature or the axial length of the eyes do not allow exact refraction of the light to form a clear retinal image then a refractive error is present.

The refractive errors are mostly due to slight variation in the axial length of the eye but may also be due to variations in the corneal curvature.

Hypermetropia (or hyperopia) (= long sight)

Myopia (= short sight)

Astigmatism.

HYPERMETROPIA (HYPEROPIA) OR LONG SIGHT

The axial length of the eye is shorter than normal. Minor amounts of hypermetropia may be overcome in young people by accommodation but moderate and high amounts require correction with spectacles (convex or positive lenses) or contact lenses to obtain a clear image.

After middle-age, when accommodation fails sufficiently, a different type of hypermetropia occurs called presbyopia.

Hypermetropia and its variant presbyopia cause the patient to have blurring of vision especially for near objects (Fig. 2.1).

MYOPIA OR SHORT SIGHT

The axial length of the eye is longer than normal. This requires correction with spectacles (concave or negative lenses) or contact lenses.

Myopia causes difficulty in seeing distant objects clearly although the near vision of myopes remains excellent (Fig. 2.2).

3

Rapid changes in refractive errors

When a refractive error changes over a short period, say, days or weeks, then an underlying cause should always be sought. Refractive errors vary only slowly over the years, except in growing children, so a rapid change should always alert the doctor or optometrist. Causes of these changes are as detailed below.

SENILE CATARACT

The nuclear sclerosis variety of cataract may progress over a short period and give rise to rapidly increasing myopia. This is because of the increasing refractive index of the lens.

DIABETES MELLITUS

With fluctuations in blood sugar level and hence aqueous sugar level the refractive index of the lens may change. An undiagnosed diabetic may become rapidly myopic over a few weeks because of the increased blood sugar level. Conversely a rapid fall in blood sugar level with treatment will cause hypermetropia and a consequent blurring of near vision. Sometimes a newly treated diabetic will complain of the increased near vision difficulty having been accustomed to the comfortable near vision and myopia of an increased blood sugar level.

Because of these rapid changes in refractive error newly treated or unstable diabetics should wait for spectacles or be given temporary ones until the diabetes has been stabilised.

EYELID LUMPS

External pressure on the eye from an eyelid or orbital swelling will induce astigmatism because of slight distortion of the cornea. Even a simple Meibomian cyst of the upper eyelid may induce a marked degree of astigmatism by this mechanism.

Fig. 3.1
Normal eye and keratoconus

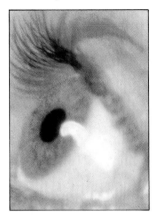

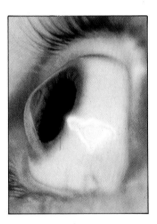

SUBLUXATION OF THE LENS

A change in position of the crystalline lens in the eye from sub-luxation will induce a rapid change in refractive error and consequent blurred vision. In a simple subluxation, when the lens is constantly moving, a change in refractive error may occur every few minutes, being hypermetropic as the lens moves backwards and myopic as the lens moves forwards. An iris or ciliary body neoplasm may cause displacement of the lens also giving similar changes in refractive error.

MIOTIC EYE DROPS

The spasm of accommodation produced by parasympathomimetic eye drops, e.g. Pilocarpine, induces an artificial myopia. Patients on miotic eye drops should only be prescribed spectacles when they are on a regular and stable dose of drops.

MYDRIATIC/CYCLOPLEGIC EYE DROPS

Relaxation of accommodation by the use of cycloplegic eye drops will be accompanied by pupil dilatation. This will induce a state of increased hypermetropia with blurring of near vision. Most patients using mydriatic/cycloplegic eye drops, e.g. Cyclopentolate 1% eye drops, will be doing so for medical reasons as in the treatment of iritis. However, they may occasionally be mistakenly applied, e.g. if old drops are available in the house; or if a friend or relative contaminates his fingers and rubs his eye accidentally. Occasionally, ephedrine nasal drops may also be inadvertently instilled into the eye by finger or skin contamination.

KERATOCONUS

The onset of keratoconus (conical cornea) may be rapid and an increase in myopia and astigmatism over a period of weeks is characteristic. Rapid variations in astigmatism should particularly alert the practitioner to the possibility of this condition occurring mostly in adolescence and early adult life (Fig. 3.1).

4

Colour vision defects

INTRODUCTION AND INCIDENCE

Colour blindness or more accurately colour defectiveness occurs in the world's population as an *inherited sex-linked recessive trait*.

The term refers to all grades of inability to distinguish or match colours but complete loss of the colour sense is extremely rare. Hence the more accurate term colour deficiency or defectiveness.

Colour deficiency occurs in all populations but is less common in Japanese, Chinese and Africans. In Western populations the incidence has been reported as 8% of males and 0.4% of females. These figures include all types varying from slight confusion between red and green colours to the complete inability to see one or more colours.

The underlying anomaly lies in the absence or deficiency of one of the photopigments in the retinal receptor cells, the cones. Complete colour blindness (achromatopsia) is a presumed absence of all the photopigments and is associated with nystagmus.

It is impossible to describe a particular colour without comparing it with other colours or coloured objects, so it is speculation as to precisely what a defective individual sees. It is known, however, that a red-green colour defective individual cannot distinguish between these colours when they are of equal brightness so possibly they are observed as shades of grey.

IMPORTANCE OF COLOUR DEFICIENCY

Modern life demands that an individual must be safe at work for his own protection and that of others. Safety is vital in a number of occupations where normal colour vision is essential such as civil and military pilots and certain ground staff, many occupations in shipping both on ships and ashore and certain railway staff. Other occupations in design, art and industry require normal colour vision for their proper pursuit.

Since early detection is desirable appropriate tests can properly be carried out with visual acuity screening in early school age.

TYPES OF COLOUR DEFECT

The types of colour defect derive their names from the three primary colours, red, green and blue, and are named after their Greek roots; *protos* (first), *deuteros* (second) and *tritos* (third) respectively. Thus:
1. Protanopia is a red (first) colour defect
2. Deuteranopia is a green (second) colour defect
3. Tritanopia is a blue (third) colour defect
When the colour defect or anomaly is only partial, they are termed:
1. Protanomalous (red partial defect)
2. Deuteranomalous (green partial defect)
3. Tritanomalous (blue partial defect)
Of the 8% of males who are colour deficient about half have a complete and half a partial defect.

The most common colour defects are for red and green (protanopia/protanomaly and deuteranopia/deuteranomaly respectively). A blue colour defect (tritanopia/tritanomaly) is rare.

ACQUIRED COLOUR DEFECTS

This occurs in many retinal and optic nerve conditions such as macular degeneration, toxic amblyopia, chronic glaucoma and diabetic retinopathy.

Senile cataracts also characteristically slowly reduce colour appreciation as they progress but normal colour vision is restored after removal of the cataracts.

TESTS FOR COLOUR VISION DEFECTS

Isochromatic charts and lantern tests form the two practical tests.

Isochromatic charts
These charts are made up of a coloured number or letter on a background of other coloured dots of equal brightness. The patient is required to identify the number or letter on the chart. The best known of these is the Ishihara test and there are other similar tests, The City University colour vision test and the H-R-R test.

The isochromatic charts are excellent quick tests for colour vision screening (Fig. 4.1, 4.2).

Fig. 4.1
The Ishihara test

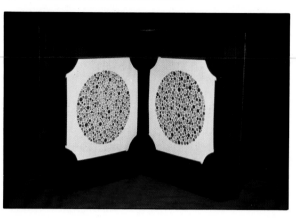

Fig. 4.2
The City University colour vision test

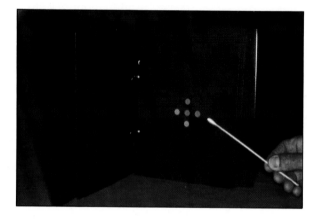

Fig. 4.3
The Giles-Archer lantern test

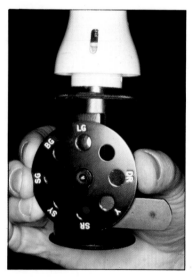

Lantern tests

A number of lantern tests are in use in aviation and the transport industries. One simple and portable version is the Giles-Archer lantern test. The patient is asked to identify a succession of coloured lights used in the transport industries as signal lights (red, green, blue-green, yellow) (Fig. 4.3).

5

Age changes in the eye

A number of physiological changes occur in the eyes and vision with increasing age. They should be recognised in order to distinguish them from pathological conditions of the eye.

The common and easily recognised changes will be described under their separate headings. They are all harmless but some may cause minor anxiety symptoms for the patient which can be allayed by a simple explanation and reassurance.

AGEING OF FUNCTION

Accommodation

Accommodation is the increase in effectivity or power of the crystalline lens by contraction of the ciliary muscle within the ciliary body (innervated by the parasympathetic fibres of the third or oculomotor nerve) which in turn relaxes the zonular fibres of the lens.

The gradual decline in accommodation causes the condition known as presbyopia and is almost inevitable in the ageing population. The decline in accommodation causes blurring of vision for close objects and is overcome by the wearing of near vision spectacles for reading, sewing, etc.

Dark adaptation

The ability of the retina to adapt to low levels of illumination occurs as a result of rhodopsin synthesis in the rod cells of the retina.

Old people adapt at a slower rate to dark conditions (dark adaptation) and hence they feel less secure in any darkened room or at night.

AGEING OF STRUCTURE

Arcus senilis of the cornea

The arcus senilis appears as a whitish ring in the periphery of the cornea with a clear zone separating it from the limbus. The appearance is due to deposition of phospholipids in the corneal periphery and can be seen in most people after late middle-age. It is harmless and does not affect vision (Fig. 5.1).

17

Fig. 5.1
Arcus senilis of the cornea

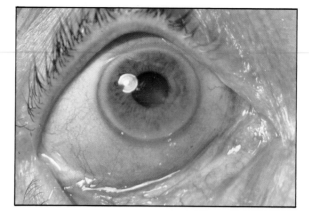

Pinguecula of the conjunctiva

Yellowish nodules on the nasal and temporal conjunctiva are frequently seen after middle-age. They consist of hyaline and lipid degenerative patches on the exposed part of the conjunctiva.

Pingueculae are harmless but may be considered a cosmetic blemish for some people, such as photographic models or film actors, and may be surgically excised if considered to be a significant blemish (Fig. 5.2).

Fig. 5.2
Pinguecula

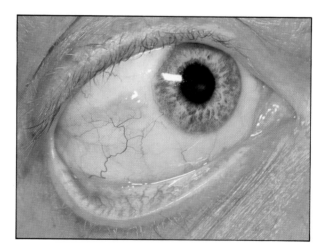

Vitreous

With age the vitreous becomes more liquid and the fine vitreous fibrils may come closer together giving rise to the appearance of condensations. These fibrillar condensations cause the symptom of floating hair-like opacities and the larger ones may be seen with the ophthalmoscope. Myopic patients may experience these 'floaters' at an earlier age than in the general population.

Particularly in middle life the condition of posterior vitreous detachment and collapse may occur. This gives rise to symptoms similar to retinal detachment (see pages 116–118) of sudden onset of floating opacities, blurred vision and flashing lights (photopsia) and gives rise to considerable anxiety. Posterior vitreous detachment is an age-related physiological collapse of the vitreous whereby liquefied vitreous enters a space formed within the vitreous internal limiting membrane, the inner layer detaching while the outer layer remains adherent to the retina.

Patients with symptoms of floaters and flashes require careful examination through a dilated pupil to distinguish between a retinal detachment or retinal tear which requires immediate treatment, and a posterior vitreous detachment which requires no treatment. The symptoms of posterior vitreous detachment usually resolve after several weeks or months. The light flashes, or photopsia, resolve when there is separation of the vitreous from the areas of retinal adhesion and the vitreous ceases to 'tug' the peripheral retina. Vitreous opacities may persist, however, indefinitely but gradually the patient learns to ignore them.

Fundus

With increasing age, arteriosclerosis of the retinal vessels occurs and this may be observed in the fundus as narrowing of the retinal arterioles and occasional variations in calibre.

Eyelids

Decrease in elastic tissue of the skin and loss of muscle tone will produce the typical appearance of age, namely loose skin folds of the eyelids or 'baggy' eyelids (blepharochalasis) with skin wrinkling.

For cosmetic reasons these loose skin folds may occasionally be surgically removed.

6

Eyelid conditions

ANATOMY AND PHYSIOLOGY

The eyelids are modified, mobile folds of skin with a firm *tarsal plate* of fibrous tissue in each to give strength and rigidity. Skin covers the outer part of the eyelid under which lies the *orbicularis oculi muscle* fibres supplied by the facial nerve (VII cranial nerve). Contraction of these fibres produces forced closure of the eyelids or 'squeezing'. Within each tarsal plate is a row of some 20 *Meibomian* glands secreting an oily sebum from openings on the eyelid margin to form an oily layer over the tear film. The inner surface of the eyelids is lined with conjunctiva, (*tarsal conjunctiva*), a mucous membrane, continuous with the conjunctiva on the anterior portion of the sclera (*bulbar conjunctiva*). Inserted into the upper portion of the tarsal plate is the *levator palpebrae superioris muscle* supplied by the oculomotor nerve (III cranial nerve). The levator muscle is responsible for the reflex act of blinking, necessary for the adequate lubrication of the surface of the eye. The eyelids, and the bony orbit, provide vital protection for the eyes from external injury (Fig. 6.1, 6.2).

Fig. 6.1
Surface markings of the eyelids

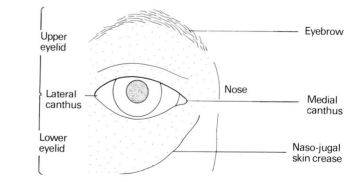

20

Fig. 6.2
Vertical section through the eyelid

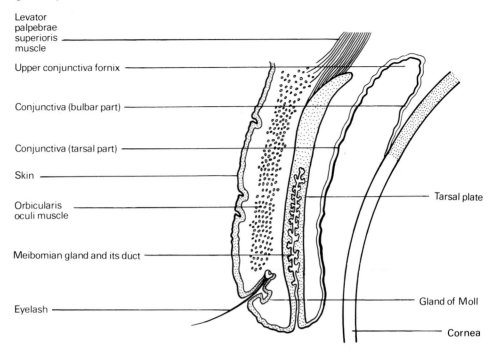

Levator palpebrae superioris muscle

Upper conjunctiva fornix

Conjunctiva (bulbar part)

Conjunctiva (tarsal part)

Skin

Orbicularis oculi muscle

Meibomian gland and its duct

Eyelash

Tarsal plate

Gland of Moll

Cornea

The following eyelid conditions will be described under their respective headings:
Congenital eyelid conditions
1. Epicanthus
2. Ptosis
Inflammatory eyelid conditions
1. Meibomian cyst (chalazion)
2. Stye
3. Blepharitis
Degenerative and malpositioning eyelid conditions
1. Cyst of Moll
2. Entropion
3. Ectropion
Neoplasms of the eyelid (benign)
1. Papilloma
2. Haemangioma
3. Xanthelasma
Neoplasms of the eyelid (malignant)
1. Basal cell carcinoma (rodent ulcer)
2. Squamous cell carcinoma

CONGENITAL EYELID CONDITIONS

Epicanthus

Many babies are born with an additional fold of skin called epicanthus which extends from the nasal aspect of the upper eyelid to the

Treatment

This is unsatisfactory and a permanent cure cannot be expected. Simple measures are helpful in controlling the inflammation and these consist of cleaning away crusts from the eyelids, often several times a day, and ensuring eyelashes do not fall into the eyes. When exacerbations occur antibiotic ointment may be applied to the eyelid margins twice a day, e.g. Oculentum Chloromycetin. However it should be emphasised that this treatment is only necessary during exacerbations as it is a chronic condition (Fig. 6.7).

Fig. 6.7
Blepharitis

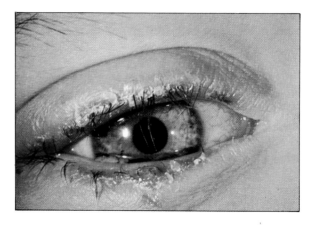

Allergic blepharitis has a rapid onset over several hours causing swelling of the eyelids and intense itching. It may occur in response to known allergies such as pollens, dust, eating shellfish or to make-up or eye drops. The swelling is usually confined to the area of contact on the skin in the case of make-up and eye drops.

Treatment

This consists of trying to remove the source of the allergy and cold compresses for the eyelids to relieve the itching and swelling (Fig. 6.8).

Fig. 6.8
Allergic blepharitis

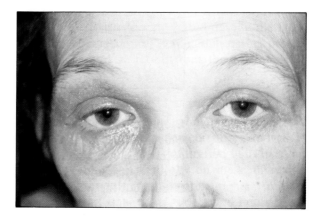

DEGENERATIVE CONDITIONS OF THE EYELIDS

Cyst of Moll

The Glands of Moll are very small sweat glands lying close to the eyelid margins. They form cystic swellings of the eyelids when obstructed. These cysts are initially small and translucent but they enlarge over many months.

Treatment
This consists of excising the cyst for cosmetic reasons or because of discomfort (Fig. 6.9).

Fig. 6.9
Cyst of Moll

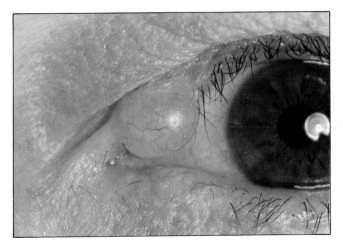

Entropion

Senile involutional entropion is a common condition occurring mainly in elderly people. The lower eyelid turns inwards causing the eyelashes to abrade the cornea and conjunctiva. This gives rise to a painful, red and discharging eye (Fig. 6.10).

Entropion may less commonly occur secondary to scarring of the tarsal conjunctiva (cicatrical entropion), or from ocular irritation from a foreign body, or keratitis (spastic entropion) because of spasm of the orbicularis oculi muscle.

Fig. 6.10
Entropion

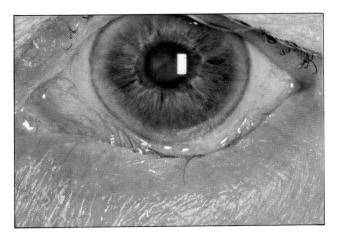

Treatment
Surgical repair is the only permanent cure for this condition and is performed as an out-patient under local anaesthetic. To relieve the patient's symptoms whilst awaiting operation the skin of the lower eyelid may be pulled down and strapped on to the cheek with narrow tape each day.

Ectropion

This is the opposite of entropion in which the lower eyelid sags downwards and turns out leaving exposed tarsal conjunctiva. The appearances are those of a reddened exposed tarsal conjunctiva and watering of the eye because the lower punctum is no longer apposed to the eye (Fig. 6.11).

Most ectropion (like entropion) occurs in elderly patients but it may occur also as a result of scarring of the eyelid skin from chemical or thermal burns or chronic eczema, or as a result of paralysis of the facial nerve (VII cranial nerve).

Treatment
Senile ectropion is treated by surgical repair of the lower eyelid performed under local anaesthetic as an out-patient.

Fig. 6.11
Ectropion. (Courtesy of the Western Ophthalmic Hospital)

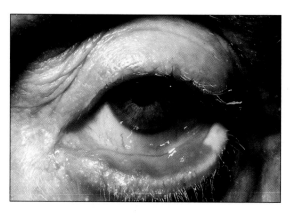

NEOPLASMS OF THE EYELID: BENIGN

Papilloma

Simple squamous papillomas are common on the eyelid as elsewhere on the skin and may be single or multiple. They are skin coloured lumps of varying size and may increase in size only very slowly or remain unchanged for many years (Fig. 6.12).

Treatment
Consists of simple excision of the papilloma either for cosmetic reasons or to relieve discomfort of the eyelid.

Fig. 6.12
Papilloma of the eyelid

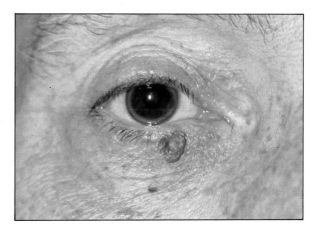

Haemangioma

These congenital benign neoplasms consist of abnormal blood vessels (cavernous or capillary haemangiomas) which are red or bluish soft swellings of the eyelid of varying size (Fig. 6.13).

Treatment
Congenital haemangiomas almost always slowly regress during the first few years of life and seldom require surgical excision.

Fig. 6.13
Haemangioma of the eyelid

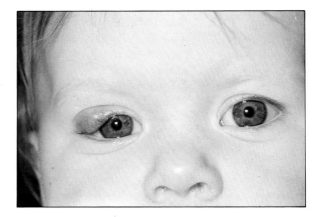

Fig. 6.14
Facial haemangioma ('port wine stain')

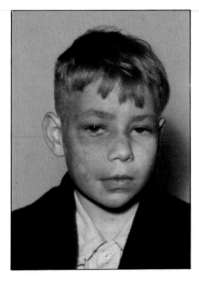

The Sturge-Weber syndrome is a condition in which a large facial capillary haemangioma ('port wine stain') is associated with meningeal and choroidal haemangiomas, and may also be associated with juvenile glaucoma (Fig. 6.14).

Xanthelasma

Yellow lipid deposits in the skin of the eyelids are called xanthelasma. These yellow, soft, flat areas commence mainly on the nasal aspects of the eyelids and gradually increase in size over several years. They are often associated with hyperlipidaemia from other causes such as diabetes mellitus, myxoedema and primary hypercholesterolaemias. Hence patients presenting with this condition should be assessed for an underlying cause (Fig. 6.15).

Treatment
Simple excision of the xanthelasma under local anaesthetic produces a good cosmetic result but recurrences may occur especially where there is an underlying systemic cause.

Fig. 6.15
Xanthelasma of the eyelids

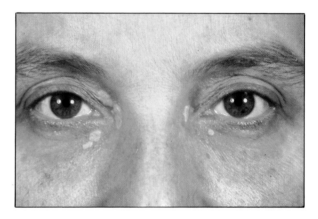

NEOPLASMS OF THE EYELID: MALIGNANT

Basal cell carcinoma (rodent ulcer)

The rodent ulcer, deriving its name from the gradual 'gnawing away' of the skin, is the most common malignant tumour of the eyelids. It commences as a small lump anywhere on the eyelid and gradually increases in size over several months until it has an ulcerated centre bordered by a raised whitish edge. The rodent ulcer is prone to bleed easily and scab over the central portion. It steadily enlarges eroding the skin and even the underlying bone as it does so. Any small lump of the skin which progressively enlarges and is prone to bleed must be regarded as a likely rodent ulcer (Fig. 6.16).

Fig. 6.16
Basal cell carcinoma—rodent ulcer—eyelid

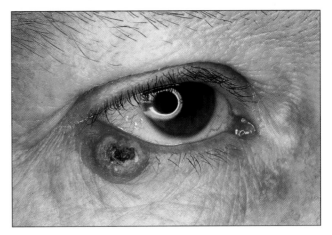

Treatment
Excision of the suspected rodent ulcer should be undertaken soon with a wide margin of normal skin being removed round the lump. Radiotherapy is also an effective treatment but biopsy of the lump beforehand of course should be undertaken to establish the diagnosis.

Squamous cell carcinoma
This is less common on the eyelid than basal cell carcinoma. An irregular progressively enlarging lump, often at the canthi, is the usual course of a squamous cell carcinoma. The lump often ulcerates and exudes fluid. Lymph node enlargement from lymphatic spread is frequent (pre-auricular and submandibular nodes) and should be carefully looked for with any eyelid lump suspected of being malignant (Fig. 6.17).

Fig. 6.17
Squamous cell carcinoma of the eyelid

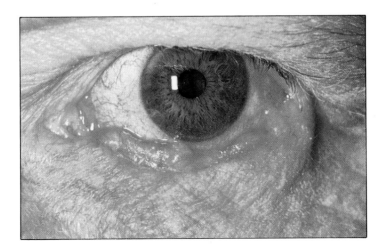

Treatment

Wide excision of the lump should be undertaken and where there is extensive eyelid involvement major plastic surgery may be required. Irradiation may also be required either on its own or in conjunction with surgery.

A note of caution should be mentioned here. In the early stages squamous cell carcinoma, of the eyelid margins in particular, (and also basal cell carcinoma) may appear as a single reddened area and thought to be blepharitis. However, blepharitis is always a bilateral chronic condition whereas carcinoma is unilateral, has a short history and is confined to one eyelid or the canthi.

7

Watering of the eyes: lacrimal disease

ANATOMY AND PHYSIOLOGY

The *lacrimal gland* lies in the upper, outer quadrant of the orbit protected by the bony orbital wall in its own fossa. Ducts from the lacrimal gland open into the upper conjunctival fornix and secrete tear fluid over the surface of the eye aided by the 'smearing' action of blinking. From the surface of the eye the tears drain into the *lacrimal punctum*, each of which is situated on the eyelid margin about one quarter of the eyelid's length from the *inner canthus*. The puncta are two very small openings draining tears into two corresponding *canaliculi* running towards the nose just beneath the skin of the eyelids. The canaliculi join a dilated portion of the lacrimal passage way called the *lacrimal sac* which lies against the bone between the orbit and the nose. The *nasolacrimal duct* completes the passage way for tear fluid running downwards and backwards in the bone into the inferior meatus of the nose (Fig. 7.1).

Fig. 7.1
Lacrimal passages

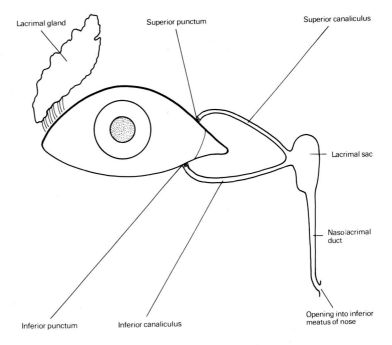

Lacrimal gland • Superior punctum • Superior canaliculus • Lacrimal sac • Nasolacrimal duct • Opening into inferior meatus of nose • Inferior punctum • Inferior canaliculus

Watering of the eyes is a frequent occurrence in any eye disease and is due to excess production of tear fluid from the lacrimal gland. There is reflex watering of the eyes (lacrimation) in any inflammatory condition such as a corneal foreign body, iritis, acute glaucoma and injury, mediated through the trigeminal nerve (V cranial nerve).

Physiological watering of the eyes may occur in particularly sensitive individuals in bright light or cold wind and also in emotional moments of sadness or laughter.

Any obstruction in the lacrimal passage ways will cause overflow of tears on to the cheek (epiphora).

Whenever watering of the eye or eyes occurs treatment should be directed to the cause.

Particular features to note when examining the lacrimal apparatus are the position and opening of the punctum, obvious overspill of tears on to the cheek, the position of the eyelids and any evidence of swelling over the lacrimal gland (lateral part of upper eyelid) or over the lacrimal sac (side of the nose).

The following conditions of the lacrimal apparatus will be considered:

Lacrimal sac, puncta and canaliculi
1. Acute dacryocystitis
2. Chronic dacryocystitis
3. Congenital nasolacrimal duct obstruction
4. Punctum and canaliculus obstruction

Lacrimal gland
1. Dacryoadenitis
2. Neoplasms

ACUTE DACRYOCYSTITIS

Acute infection of the lacrimal sac will almost always occur where there is pre-existing chronic obstruction or infection. Consequently there will be a long history, often of several years duration, of watering of the eye due to obstruction of the nasolacrimal duct.

The *symptom* of acute dacryocystitis is rapid onset of a painful swelling at the side of the nose ('the inner canthus of the eye'). The characteristic *sign* is a reddened, tender, tense swelling between the side of the nose and just below the inner canthus. Watering and discharge from the eye usually occur.

Treatment
Systemic antibiotics are required (e.g. ampicillin or flucloxacillin 250 mg four times a day for 7 days). When the acute inflammation has subsided a mucocoele (collection of mucus in the dilated lacrimal sac) may remain with constant regurgitation of mucus upwards into the conjunctiva. When this and recurrent dacryocystitis occurs a permanent cure can only be achieved by the surgical operation of dacryocystorhinostomy (DCR). In this operation a new passage way for tears is made joining the lacrimal sac directly

to the nasal cavity, thus by-passing the obstructed nasolacrimal duct (Fig. 7.2).

Fig. 7.2
Acute dacryocystitis

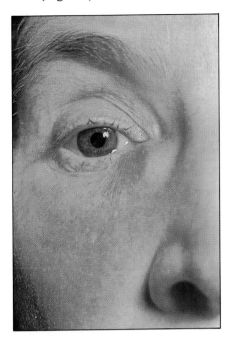

Chronic dacryocystitis

Long standing watering of the eyes in the elderly patient is a common occurrence. It is due to obstruction of the nasolacrimal duct from chronic infection. The *symptom* experienced by the patient is overspill of tears on to the cheeks especially in cold winds. The *signs* to be noted are the position of the puncta and the absence of any inflammation or swelling. The diagnosis may be confirmed by gently syringing saline through the lower punctum and canaliculus, after instillation of local anaesthetic drops (amethocaine or benoxinate). If the patient can feel saline in his nasopharynx then the lacrimal passage way must be clear. If not and it returns via the upper punctum then this indicates obstruction of the nasolacrimal duct (Fig. 7.3).

Fig. 7.3
Syringing the nasolacrimal duct

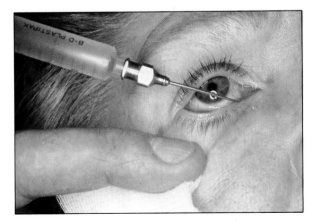

Treatment

Mild degrees of watering due to nasolacrimal duct obstruction in the elderly are best left untreated. A simple explanation of this harmless condition will allay the anxiety of the patient and allow him to accept this minor disability once the diagnosis has been made. Sometimes zinc sulphate 0.25% eye drops produce slight symptomatic relief.

Severe watering of the eyes can be very distressing, producing erythema and dryness of the skin of the cheeks with blurring of vision. The only effective treatment in these circumstances is the operation of dacryocystorhinostomy which by-passes the obstructed nasolacrimal duct by anastomosing the mucosa lining the lacrimal sac with that of the nasal passage way through a new opening in the bone.

Congenital obstruction of the nasolacrimal duct

Unilateral or bilateral sticky eyes in babies during the first nine months of life are frequently caused by late opening (or canalisation) of the lower end of the nasolacrimal duct. Delayed opening of the duct may be recognised by sticky and watering eyes in the baby from birth.

Treatment

A culture of the conjunctival discharge should first be taken to identify any bacterial infection.

Antibiotic eye drops such as Chloromycetin, are instilled two or three times a day and the parents are instructed in cleaning the eyelids with cotton wool and water, keeping them free of mucus, also two or three times a day. This treatment will need to be continued until the expected spontaneous resolution occurs before the age of 8 or 9 months, although the antibiotic eye drops may be discontinued after about a month.

Spontaneous opening of the lower end of the nasolacrimal duct(s) may be expected in most babies but when watering and stickiness of the eyes continues beyond 8 or 9 months, natural resolution is unlikely. When symptoms persist after 8 or 9 months probing of the duct should be performed under general anaesthetic in order to open the portion at the lower end obstructed by fibrous tissue.

Punctum and canaliculus obstruction

Congenital absence or incomplete development of the punctum and canaliculus will cause the same symptoms as a congenitally obstructed nasolacrimal duct, namely, watering and stickiness of the eye. However they are not common and abnormalities of the punctum can be recognised by simple inspection of the eyelid margins.

Treatment

This usually consists of an extensive canaliculus reconstruction operation. More commonly punctum and canaliculus obstruction are caused as a complication of chronic conjunctivitis in adults especially viral conjunctivitis such as herpes simplex conjunctivitis and trachoma, or as an accompaniment of mucocutaneous disease (pemphigus, ocular pemphigoid, erythema multiforme—Stevens-Johnson syndrome) (Fig. 7.4).

Fig. 7.4
Ocular pemphigoid

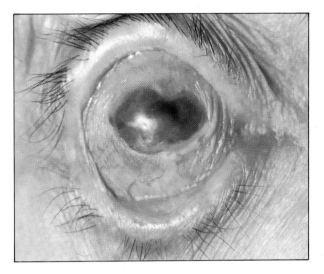

LACRIMAL GLAND

Dacryoadenitis

Dacryoadenitis is inflammation of the lacrimal gland. The *symptoms* are swelling and tenderness of the lateral aspect of the upper eyelid often with epiphora. The *signs* are a tender swelling on the lateral aspect of the upper eyelid with erythema of the overlying skin. Gently raising the upper eyelid will reveal the enlarged, sometimes discharging, lacrimal gland. The pre-auricular lymph nodes may also be enlarged (Fig. 7.5, 7.6).

Dacryoadenitis is most common in young people and may be caused by:

1. *Acute infections*, such as by staphylococci or Haemophilus influenzae bacteria which may be blood-borne but may also be introduced by injuries to the lacrimal gland.

2. *Chronic infections*, may be tubercular in origin and in these patients there may be other signs, e.g. pulmonary tuberculosis.

3. *Mumps*, a virus infection occurring mainly in children which causes enlargement of the lacrimal and salivary glands and usually resolves over a few days.

4. *Sarcoidosis*, which frequently involves the lacrimal glands causing a chronic dacryoadenitis. There may be other signs of sarcoidosis such as enlarged salivary glands, pulmonary and skin changes.

Fig. 7.5
Acute dacryoadenitis

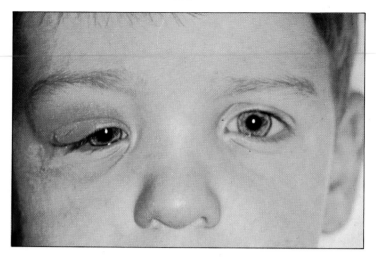

Fig. 7.6
Inflamed lacrimal gland

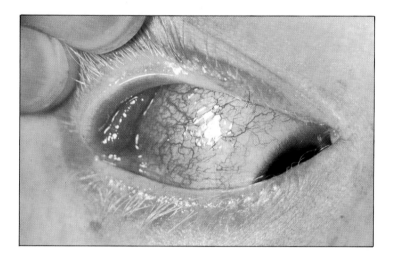

Treatment
The treatment of dacryoadenitis is directed at the cause in each case. Where a precise diagnosis of a chronic dacryoadenitis is not possible with clinical evidence alone, it is sometimes necessary to perform a surgical biopsy of the enlarged gland for microscopic examination.

Neoplasms of the lacrimal gland
Tumours of the lacrimal gland are uncommon but occur mainly in the middle-aged. The *clinical features* are progressive enlargement of the gland which can be felt through the upper eyelid as a hard irregular mass. This occurs gradually over several months and as a result the eye becomes displaced downwards and inwards from the external pressure.

The majority of lacrimal gland neoplasms are mixed tumours and adenoidcystic carcinomas, but occasionally reticulosis.

Mixed tumours, so called because they contain mesenchymal and epithelial elements, affect middle-age people and are slow-growing often with a history of 12 months. Treatment is by local surgical excision.

Adenoidcystic carcinomas also present in middle-age but the history of gland swelling is shorter, over a few weeks. Treatment is by radiotherapy, or radical surgical excision for the locally invasive tumours.

Lymphoma or lymphosarcoma of the lacrimal gland is usually associated with widespread reticulosis. Treatment is usually by radiotherapy or chemotherapy.

8

Red (inflamed) eyes

ANATOMY

It is helpful to recall that the anterior portion of the eye has two separate blood supplies, namely the conjunctival and ciliary vessels. The conjunctival arteries are numerous small branches from the *eyelid arterial arcades* and the anterior ciliary arteries. They have numerous corresponding veins providing venous blood drainage.

The anterior ciliary arteries are continuations of the paired arteries running forwards in the four rectus muscles and they can easily be seen in normal eyes. They penetrate the sclera to supply blood to the ciliary body and iris, also sending off small branches which join the conjunctival vessels. Venous drainage is by similar ciliary veins.

The two long posterior ciliary arteries are branches of the ophthalmic artery and penetrate the sclera either side of the optic nerve and then pass forwards in the space between choroid and sclera to anastomose with the anterior ciliary arteries in the ciliary body to form the *major arterial circle of the iris* (Fig. 8.1, 8.2).

Figs 8.1 and 8.2
Blood supply to anterior portion of eye and eyelids

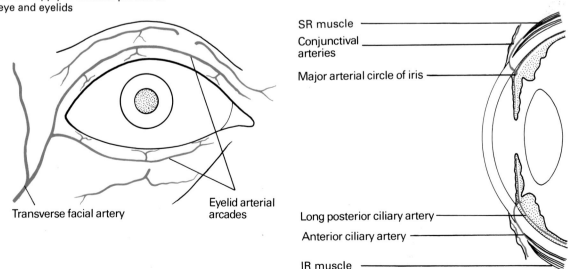

Transverse facial artery

Eyelid arterial arcades

SR muscle

Conjunctival arteries

Major arterial circle of iris

Long posterior ciliary artery

Anterior ciliary artery

IR muscle

Conditions of the iris, ciliary body and cornea therefore cause dilatation of the ciliary vessels and this is called *ciliary hyperaemia or injection.*

Conditions of the conjunctiva cause dilatation of the conjunctival vessels, called *conjunctival hyperaemia or injection.*

Inflammation of the anterior portion of the eyes causes the striking reddened appearance. The conditions responsible for this are grouped according to whether conjunctival or ciliary vessels are dilated:

Conjunctival vessel hyperaemia (injection): Conjunctivitis.

Ciliary vessel hyperaemia (injection): Iritis, keratitis, acute glaucoma.

SUMMARY OF SYMPTOMS AND SIGNS OF CAUSES OF RED EYES

	Symptoms	Signs
Conjunctivitis	Red eyes Bilateral (usually) Gritty feeling Stickiness	Conjunctival hyperaemia Swollen eyelids Mucoid discharge
Iritis	Red eye Unilateral (usually) Lacrimation Photophobia Blurred vision Pain	Reduced vision Ciliary injection Constricted pupil Flare in AC KP
Keratitis	Red eye Unilateral (usually) Lacrimation Photophobia Blurred vision Pain	Reduced vision Ciliary injection Localised corneal opacification
Acute glaucoma	Red eye Unilateral (usually) Lacrimation Photophobia Blurred vision Pain Haloes	Reduced vision Ciliary injection Corneal oedema (cloudy) Pupil half dilated and oval Raised ocular tension

CONJUNCTIVITIS

Inflammation of the conjunctiva, a mucous membrane, is called conjunctivitis. There are several causal agents and they may be listed as follows:

1. *Bacterial infections*, especially staphylococcus, *Haemophilus influenzae* and streptococcus

2. *Viral infections*, especially Herpes simplex, adenovirus and *Chlamydia trachomatis* (TRIC agent)
3. *Trauma*, especially chemicals and ultraviolet energy irradiation (see Ch. 9)
4. *Dry eyes (conjunctivitis sicca)*, due to lack of tear secretion

Symptoms
1. Condition is usually bilateral
2. Sensation of grittiness or 'sandy' feeling
3. Stickiness of the eyelids
4. Reddened appearance of the eyes
5. In severe cases the eyelids are swollen
6. Vision is not affected
7. Itching—an additional symptom of allergic conjunctivitis
8. In cases of trauma there will be a history of exposure to ultraviolet light or chemicals

Signs
1. Conjunctival hyperaemia (Fig. 8.3)
2. Mucus discharge on the lids with crusting of the eyelashes
3. Eyelid swelling

Fig. 8.3
Acute conjunctivitis

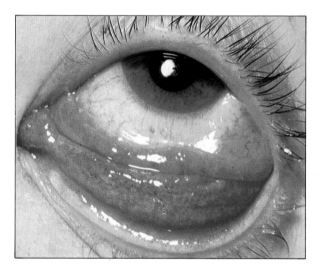

Treatment
In all cases of conjunctivitis, even when simple allergy seems likely, a swab is taken for *bacterial culture*. (Viral cultures and conjunctival cell scrapings are also taken in some situations but this is rather specialised work.) Cleaning the crusting on the eyelids every few hours with cotton wool soaked in tepid water aids comfort. Antibiotic eye drops are instilled initially every two hours. Chloramphenicol (Chloromycetin) is most widely used and only changed if the culture shows the bacterium is not sensitive. Tinted spectacles may relieve discomfort from bright light and provide a cosmetic 'shield' for the reddened eyes.

Conjunctivitis usually settles in three or four days on antibiotic eye drops. If it does not then it means the causative organisms is likely to be viral, in which case symptoms may persist for many weeks, and requires specialist treatment using anti-viral eye drops and ointments (Idoxuridine 0.5%, Trifluorothymidine, Acyclovir 3%).

Pre-auricular lymphadenopathy and conjunctival follicles are common features of conjunctivitis caused by adenovirus, Herpes simplex and *Chlamydia trachomatis* in the acute stage. Follicles are fine (about 1 mm) rounded collections of lymphoid tissue, mostly in the inferior conjunctival fornix.

Neonatal conjunctivitis (*ophthalmia neonatorum*) deserves special mention because of its severity and potential to progress to keratitis with secondary corneal scarring. Conjunctivitis arises from contact with an infected birth canal. Typically conjunctivitis caused by *Neiserria gonorrhoeae* is present from 2–4 days whereas other bacterial causes and *Chlamydia trachomatis* occur a few days later from 2–14 days. Bacterial cultures and conjunctival scrapings of cells should be performed on presentation (the conjunctival cell scrapings demonstrate inclusion bodies with Giemsa staining in *Chlamydia trachomatis*) and treatment commenced at once.

Chronic perennial allergic conjunctivitis and vernal conjunctivitis

Special mention should be made of the additional symptom of itching and additional sign of papillae on the tarsal conjunctiva in allergic conjunctivitis. The papillae are characteristic and observed by everting the upper eyelid (Fig. 8.4).

Fig. 8.4
Vernal conjunctivitis showing papillae upper tarsal conjunctiva

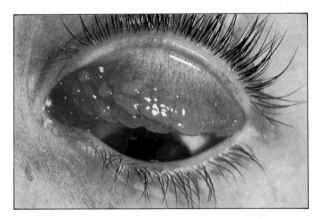

In chronic perennial allergic conjunctivitis the patients are usually adult with a history of months or years of persistent itching, discomfort, watering and light sensitivity of the eyes.

In vernal conjunctivitis the patients are characteristically young, frequently children and often have a history of additional atopic disease (asthma, hay fever and eczema).

Specific anti-allergic treatment is in the form of appropriate steroid eye drops (prednisolone, betamethasone) for the most severe cases and sodium cromoglycate 2% eye drops (Opticrom) and antazoline sulphate (Otrivine-Antistine) for the milder cases. Treatment may need to be continued for months and even years in many young people until natural remission occurs.

Dry eyes (conjunctivitis sicca)

This gives rise to progressive dry and gritty eyes, more commonly in women than men, after middle-age. It may also be associated with a similar drying of the mouth and throat. When associated with rheumatoid arthritis, conjunctivitis sicca is called Sjögren's syndrome.

The cause of the dry eyes is a progressive, possibly senile, atrophy of the lacrimal gland with reduced tear secretion as measured with Schirmer's test using thin filter paper strips. There is hyperaemia of the conjunctiva. Symptoms usually wax and wane over the months.

Fig. 8.5
Schirmer's tear flow test

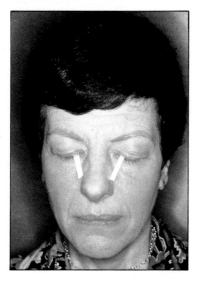

Schirmer's test

A thin (4 mm wide) strip of filter paper is placed in the lower conjunctival fornix of each eye folded over the eyelid margin. These are left in place for 5 minutes. The extent of wetting of the paper strip is then measured. A normal wetting length of the paper is more than 12 mm and in dry eyes measurements of 1–5 mm are usual (Fig. 8.5).

Treatment

Constant daily use of replacement artificial tear drops (such as Hypromellose, Adsorbotear, Liquifilm tears and Isopto Plain eye drops) will be necessary for the rest of the patient's life. Instillation as often as 1–2 hourly may be required with severe symptoms. Surgical occlusion of the four lacrimal puncta may give relief of the symptoms by retaining on the surface of the eyes the existing tears.

Lubricating eye ointments (such as Oculentum Lacri-Lube) may also be used, either combined with artificial tear drops or as an alternative. The eye ointment has the benefit of having a longer effect but temporarily blurs the vision.

Chronic conjunctivitis

More accurately described as a 'conjunctivopathy' this common but mild and harmless condition causes endless anxiety amongst patients. Mild grittiness and intermittent redness of the eyes may occur for years. The signs are minimal with just slight hyperaemia and often minute calcium deposits in the conjunctiva (concretions) observable as white specks on the tarsal conjunctiva.

Treatment

The treatment of this chronic condition is not very effective but soothing astringent eye drops, of which there are many, may be prescribed whenever the discomfort is excessive. General measures such as avoiding conditions of smoke, dust and wind are likely to be more effective.

IRITIS

The iris, ciliary body and choroid are one continuous layer called the uveal tract and because of their vascularity intraocular inflammation predominates in these structures.

Inflammation of the iris (iritis) invariably occurs with that of the ciliary body (cyclitis) so the terms iritis, iridocyclitis and anterior uveitis are interchangeable for practical purposes. The inflammation within iris tissues is likely to be due to an antigen-antibody reaction in a previously sensitised iris. The seronegative arthropathies (such as Still's disease, Reiter's disease and Behçet's disease in particular) are associated with iritis. *Histocompatibility antigens* (HLA) have been associated with iritis especially HLA-B27. Precisely how this mechanism occurs is not fully understood, but explains the recurrent nature of iritis. The known conditions associated with iritis are:
1. Sarcoidosis
2. Reiter's disease
3. Ankylosing spondylitis
4. Still's disease (Juvenile Rheumatoid Arthritis) in children
5. Behçet's disease
6. Tuberculosis
7. Syphilis
8. Leprosy

There may be a past history of any of these conditions in a patient presenting with iritis indicating a possible association. *Investigations* for a patient with a first attack of iritis should include full blood count; X-rays of sacro-iliac joints and chest; serological tests for syphilis; Mantoux test, proceeding to further investigations if indicated.

However, it should be stressed that the cause of iritis is seldom established.

Symptoms
1. Rapid blurring of vision in one (or both) eye(s) over hours or days
2. Redness of the eye
3. Aching pain in the eye
4. Photophobia
5. Watering of the eye

Signs
1. Reduced visual acuity
2. Ciliary vessel hyperaemia

3. Pupil constriction—because of inflammatory spasm of the iris sphincter muscle
4. Pupil irregularity—*posterior synechiae* are adhesions between the iris and lens and may lead to a secondary glaucoma (Fig. 8.7)
5. Flare and cells in the anterior chamber—protein exudate and inflammatory cells respectively may be seen with a focused light in the anterior chamber (Fig. 8.6)

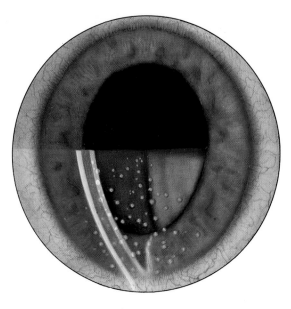

Fig. 8.6
Painting of flare and keratitic precipitates (KP) on posterior corneal surface in iritis

6. Keratitic precipitates (KP)—the inflammatory cells circulating in the aqueous may be deposited on the posterior surface of the cornea in blobs (Fig. 8.6)
7. Swelling of the eyelids

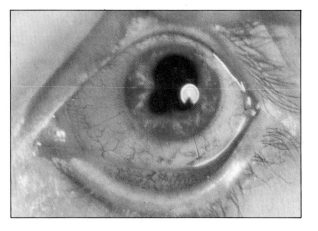

Fig. 8.7
Posterior synechiae in iritis

Treatment
Once the diagnosis of iritis has been established treatment should

Fig. 8.8
Extensive KP in iritis

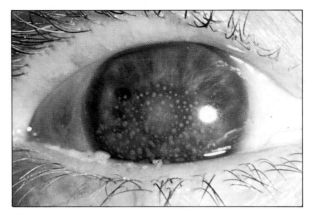

be initiated. Mydriatic eye drops (Atropine 1%, Cyclopentolate 1%, Tropicamide 1%, Hyoscine ¼% drops) are instilled two or three times a day to dilate the pupil and thus prevent posterior synechiae. Simultaneously steroid eye drops are instilled (prednisolone, betamethasone or dexamethasone drops) every 2 hours initially. The choice of the mydriatic and steroid eye drops depends on the severity of the iritis. Treatment should be continued as long as signs persist which may be as long as several months. The frequency of instillation of steroid drops may be gradually reduced as the iritis settles.

Any underlying disease should receive in addition specific treatment as required.

KERATITIS

This term covers any inflammation of the cornea. Since the cornea is exposed constantly during the waking day it is not surprising that externally induced infection occurs fairly commonly.

Keratitis initially produces a localised *oedema* of the cornea, rapidly followed by *infiltration* of inflammatory cells, hence the invariable sign of a localised corneal opacity. With long standing keratitis *vascularisation* of the cornea and abscess formation occur (Fig. 8.9).

Fig. 8.9
Corneal abscess: note white area of abscess of inflammatory cells. (Courtesy of the Western Ophthalmic Hospital)

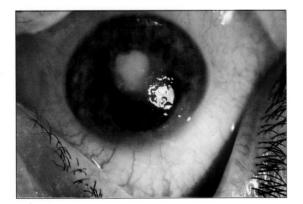

The usual organisms causing keratitis are bacteria such as staphylococci, streptococci and *Chlamydia trachomatis* and viruses such as Herpes simplex, adenovirus and Herpes zoster.

Symptoms
1. Rapid blurring of vision in one (or both) eye(s)
2. Redness of the eye
3. Aching pain in the eye
4. Photophobia
5. Watering of the eye

Signs
1. Reduced visual acuity
2. Ciliary vessel hyperaemia
3. Swelling of eyelids
4. Localised corneal opacity. This is the most important and distinctive sign of keratitis. The appearance of the localised corneal opacity depends on the cause of the keratitis.

Herpes simplex keratitis
There is a characteristic dendritic ulcer visible on the cornea which is easier to see if a staining drop of fluorescein or bengal rose is instilled (Fig. 8.10, 8.11).

Fig. 8.10
Dendritic ulcer of cornea (stained with fluorescein)

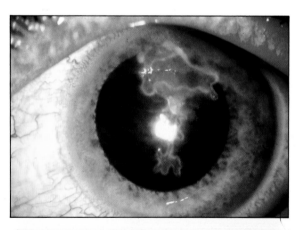

Fig. 8.11
Dendritic ulcer of cornea (stained with bengal rose)

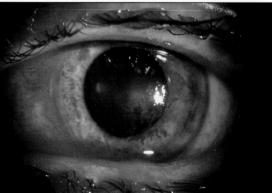

The ulcer may progress to involve the deeper (stromal) layers of the cornea, in which case the whole cornea becomes variably opaque. Treatment of a dendritic ulcer, or its deeper form, is by anti-viral eye drops or ointment of Acyclovir (Zovirax), every 2 hours and is likely to be required for several weeks (Fig. 8.12).

Fig. 8.12
Deep stromal keratitis in herpes simplex

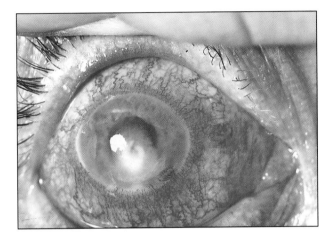

Adenovirus keratitis

Adenovirus keratoconjunctivitis often occurs in epidemics and medical personnel must pay particular attention to hand washing after examining an infected patient.

The particular features are the intense follicular conjunctivitis with spots of corneal infiltrate. These spots may take a year or more to clear. Treatment is by anti-viral eye drops or ointment (Acyclovir) 2–3 hourly and may be required for several weeks (Fig. 8.13).

Fig. 8.13
Adenovirus keratitis showing spot corneal opacities and ciliary hyperaemia

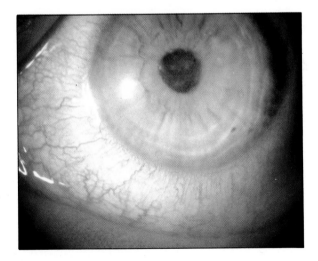

Trachoma keratitis

Endemic in many parts of the world where it is caused by the *Chlamydia trachomatis* organism and is spread by direct contact under poor hygienic conditions. A characteristic vascularised opacity in the upper cornea occurs (*pannus*) which may spread to involve the whole cornea. Simultaneously a severe conjunctivitis occurs so that trachoma is always a kerato-conjunctivitis in the early stages (Fig. 8.14).

Fig. 8.14
Pannus in trachomatous keratitis

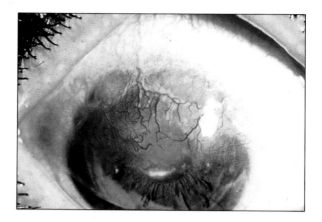

With the progression of the corneal opacification, tarsal conjunctival scarring also occurs which may cause entropion of the eyelids and *trichiasis* (ingrowing eyelashes) which in turn causes further damage to the cornea (Fig. 8.15).

Fig. 8.15
Trichiasis and corneal scarring following trachomatous keratitis

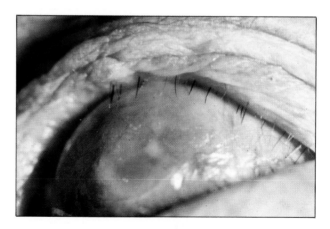

Treatment

Treatment of trachoma keratitis is by using tetracycline or sulphonamide eye ointment instilled 3-hourly during the day and may be required for many months.

If scarring of the cornea occurs following keratitis to an extent that vision is severely affected a corneal transplant (keratoplasty) operation may be necessary.

Herpes zoster ophthalmicus

Herpes zoster ophthalmicus ('shingles') is the result of infection by the varicella virus (chickenpox virus) of the trigeminal nerve (V cranial nerve) ganglion. The majority of cases are in the elderly and may occur when there is impaired immunity, such as when there is concurrent neoplasia. The condition is characterised by a *unilateral* skin rash over the forehead and usually the side of the nose which corresponds to the skin distribution of the trigeminal nerve. Vesicles over the affected skin with pain are followed by scabbing of the dried up vesicles after a number of days. Gradually the scabs fall off over a few weeks leaving some skin scarring. The pain of post-herpes zoster neuralgia on the side of the head may persist for many months or years. Analgesic tablets are taken as required to relieve the pain.

During the acute phase of skin vesicles treatment is with antiviral skin cream (Acyclovir/Zovirax) for 4–5 days in the more severe cases. Moderate and severe cases and immunocompromised patients benefit from additional systemic Acyclovir tablets (or suspension) 800 mg five times daily for 5 days. Systemic treatment is reported to halt vesiculation, speed healing and improve neuralgia pain both during the attack and later (post-herpetic).

Complications of Herpes zoster ophthalmicus are iritis and keratitis which are treated with steroid eye drops (such as betamethasone). A low grade iritis may continue for many months after the acute stage and reduced corneal sensation may remain permanently (Fig. 8.16).

Fig. 8.16
Herpes zoster ophthalmicus

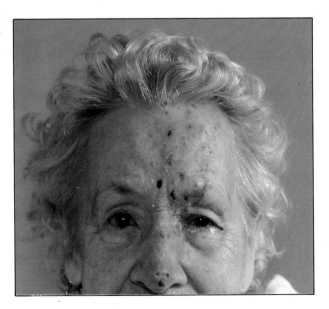

ACUTE GLAUCOMA

See Chapter 12 on glaucoma.

OTHER CAUSES

Other causes of red eyes are listed below.

Pterygium

Exposure to hot, dry and dusty conditions in many parts of the world, e.g. India, Africa and Australia causes a thickening and in-growth of the palpebral conjunctiva on to the cornea. Minor degrees of pterygium formation are extremely common and require no treatment but where growth over the cornea occurs over months and years surgical removal is indicated (Fig. 8.17).

Fig. 8.17
Pterygium

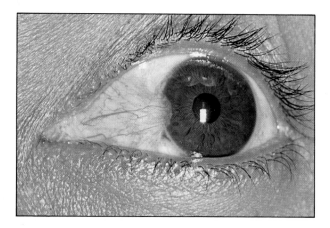

Episcleritis

This slightly raised and localised area of hyperaemia of the episcleral vessels, close to the corneal margin, causes minor discomfort and is often noted only by chance when a patient observes redness of the eye. Its cause is unknown and usually settles without treatment in a few days. Recurrence is frequent (Fig. 8.18).

Fig. 8.18
Episcleritis

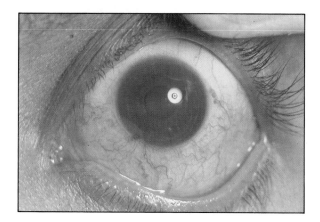

Scleritis

Inflammation of the deep layers of the sclera is less common than episcleritis but potentially serious. The patient experiences a dull aching pain with intense localised ciliary hyperaemia over one part of the eye. This may spread to involve the whole sclera and usually continues for some years (Fig. 8.19).

Fig. 8.19
Scleritis

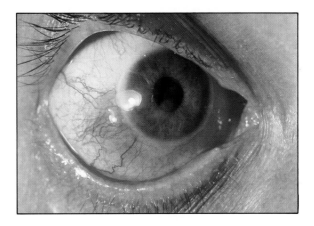

Systemic conditions associated with scleritis are rheumatoid arthritis, in particular, and the collagen diseases lupus erythematosus and polyarteritis nodosa.

Treatment is by steroid eye drops varying in strength and frequency according to the severity of the condition. Systemic steroid therapy may also be necessary in the more severe causes. Treatment, however, may be unsatisfactory.

9

Eye injuries and first aid

Eye injuries are dramatic and invariably produce considerable emotional upset for the patient. Whenever possible advice should be provided to prevent them occurring in industrial and social environments.

PREVENTION OF EYE INJURIES

Industry and building
Adequate protective spectacles or visors should be worn to prevent foreign body, irradiation (especially ultraviolet and infra-red radiation) and chemical injuries to the eyes.

Transport
The wearing of seat belts prevents most of the severe eye injuries caused by an unrestrained occupant being thrown through the windscreen. Laminated rather than toughened glass windscreens are preferable in motor vehicles as this markedly reduces splintering.

Fig. 9.1
Protective eyewear for racket sports

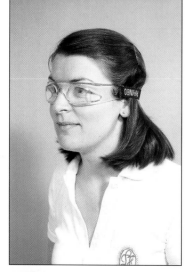

Sports
Plastic spectacle lenses or contact lenses should be worn by all sportsmen and sportswomen where spectacles are required to correct a refractive error. Myopic patients should be discouraged from boxing because of their probable greater incidence of retinal detachment. Skiers and yachtsmen should wear appropriate tinted spectacles or goggles to prevent ultraviolet light irradiation eye injuries ('snow blindness'). In some racket sports, especially squash, racketball and rackets, eye protection is advisable because of the high velocity and size of the ball and because of the close proximity of players making racket injuries more likely (Fig. 9.1).

Other occasions
The sun should never be looked at directly with or without tinted spectacles because of the risk of retinal (macular) burns. This applies especially at the time of a sun's eclipse. Do-it-yourself handymen should use protective goggles or spectacles (polycarbonate) when using power drills or heavy hammers.

Fig. 9.2
Simple essentials for eye first aid

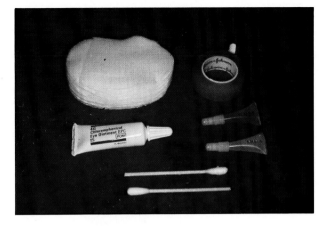

FIRST AID EQUIPMENT

The simplest first aid equipment suitable for factory, sports grounds or home should contain the following (Fig. 9.2):

1. Cotton buds (for removing superficial foreign bodies and stick for everting the eyelid)
2. Eye pads
3. Tape (for holding eyepad in place)
4. Single dose eye drops, e.g. amethocaine or benoxinate (local anaesthetic); Chloromycetin (chloramphenicol); fluorescein (for staining the cornea)
5. Antibiotic eye ointment, e.g. Chloromycetin or Neomycin
6. Torch (for illumination)

Single dose ampoules of local anaesthetic, fluorescein and antibiotic eye drops are the most suitable in order to retain a supply of sterile eye drops which can be discarded after use. The local anaesthetic drops anaesthetise the superficial cornea and conjunctiva. The antibiotic drops or ointment are for instillation after removing superficial foreign bodies and the fluorescein drops are used when necessary to detect corneal abrasions as they stain the damaged areas bright green.

Sharp instruments for removing foreign bodies should be avoided. Cotton buds will adequately remove any superficial foreign body on the eye after instillation of local anaesthetic. After any treatment to the eye an eye pad may be applied, held in place with narrow adhesive tape.

In factories where chemicals are used running water taps should be readily accessible for irrigation of the eyes.

Eversion of the eyelid
This simple technique should be employed whenever a foreign body is suspected. The patient is asked to look down, the cotton bud handle (or matchstick) is placed horizontally on the upper

eyelid, the eyelashes held and the eyelid gently turned over the cotton bud handle (Fig. 9.3, 9.4).

By this technique foreign bodies, lodged under the upper eyelid, may be removed.

Fig. 9.3
Eversion of eyelid 1

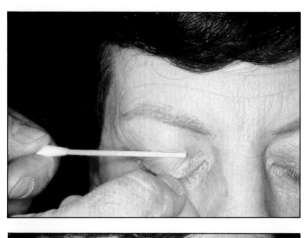

Fig. 9.4
Eversion of eyelid 2

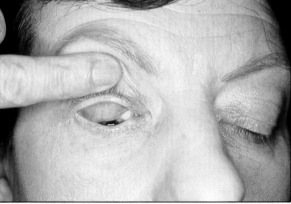

ORBITAL INJURIES

A severe concussion blow to the orbital region by a heavy object or fist usually causes considerable periorbital swelling and bruising which may be so extensive that it is difficult to open the eyelids, even forcibly, to examine the eye. Bleeding into the orbit from a blow will cause protrusion of the eye (proptosis).

'*Blow out*' *fractures* of the orbital floor should be suspected whenever there is any severe periorbital swelling and bruising from a blow. The fracture is a break in the floor of the orbit and can be recognised clinically by:

1. The history of a blow to the orbit
2. Enophthalmos, due to soft orbital tissues protruding through the fractured orbital floor causing the eye to sink back in the orbit

3. Diplopia on looking upwards because of tethering of the inferior rectus muscle in the fracture line. The tethered inferior rectus muscle 'fixes' the eye so that on attempted upward gaze the eye fails to elevate

4. Anaesthesia of the skin of the lower eyelid and cheek because of damage to the infraorbital nerve

5. Bruising and sometimes surgical emphysema of the eyelids due to escape of air from associated fractures of the ethmoid sinuses

An X-ray of the orbit is essential in any patient with periorbital bruising from a blow to detect a 'blow out' or other orbital wall fracture. Providing damage to the eye itself has not taken place it is safe to observe the patient to await settling of the periorbital bruising and very frequently the tethered inferior rectus muscle releases itself in 7–10 days. Only if diplopia continues for a few weeks after the injury is it necessary to release the tethered inferior rectus muscle and repair the orbital floor by surgical operation (Fig. 9.5).

Fig. 9.5
Orbital and subconjunctival haemorrhage

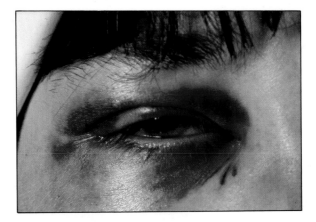

EYELID INJURIES

Lacerations of the eyelid from sharp objects should be cleaned and sutured as soon as possible taking particular care to repair the tissue layers very carefully to prevent distortion of the eyelids. Any laceration on the medial quarter of the lower eyelid should receive particular attention because of the danger of severance of the lower canaliculus.

EYE INJURIES

Subconjunctival haemorrhage

Bleeding into the subconjunctival tissue can occur from even a trivial injury. The bright red appearance localised to one area of the conjunctiva is characteristic. No treatment is required provided there is no other injured tissue. The haemorrhage spontaneously resolves over about 10–14 days (Fig. 9.5).

Fig. 9.6
Corneal foreign body

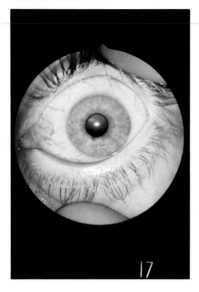

Conjunctival and corneal foreign bodies

Small particles may blow on to the surface of the eye and cause an intense pricking sensation, redness and watering of the eye. With a good light and also everting the upper eyelid the foreign body can be detected on the surface of the cornea or conjunctiva.

Treatment

Local anaesthetic drops should be instilled and the foreign body gently removed with a cotton bud. Any associated corneal abrasion can be detected using fluorescein drops. Antibiotic ointment is then instilled and an eye pad applied for a few hours (Fig. 9.6).

Corneal abrasions

A glancing blow to the eye from a finger nail or twig, for example, causes sloughing away of the affected surface corneal epithelium. Almost at once the eye becomes very painful, watery, red and photophobic. The diagnosis may readily be made by using fluorescein to detect the corneal abrasion. Exposure to ultraviolet light as in arc welders ('arc eye') produces similar severe pain in both eyes.

Treatment

Antibiotic eye ointment is instilled (such as Chloromycetin) and a firm pad applied for 24 hours ensuring the eyelids are closed behind the pad. The pad is renewed in 24 hours and most small corneal abrasions (including the multiple tiny corneal abrasions of ultraviolet light exposure) are healed in 48 hours (Fig. 9.7).

Fig. 9.7
Corneal abrasion stained with fluorescein

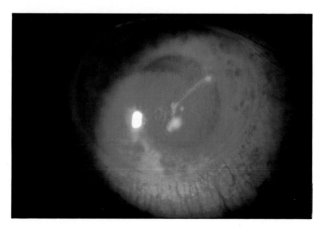

Recurrent corneal abrasion is the name given to a repeated painful eye, weeks or months after the original injury and usually presents in the early morning after awakening. It is due to recurrent break down of the originally damaged corneal epithelium and mimics the signs and symptoms of the original abrasion. When such recurrent abrasions occur nightly lubricating ointment (such as Lacri-Lube: petrolatum mineral oil) may prevent these episodes.

Chemical injuries

Whenever chemicals *of any description* are splashed into the eyes *immediate* immersion of the eyes in water is vital and washing the eyes liberally, preferably in running water, should be continued for as long as 20 minutes. Specialist treatment should then be sought at once.

Hyphaema (haemorrhage into the anterior chamber)

A concussion injury to the eye from a blow, say from a fist, explosion or any heavy object may cause haemorrhage into the anterior chamber (between the cornea and iris) from rupture of iris blood vessels.

There is immediate severe pain and blurring of vision and in a few minutes the eye becomes hyperaemic. Examination reveals blood in the anterior chamber which forms a 'fluid level' and obscures a view of the iris and pupil. Rest in bed in hospital or home is necessary because of the danger of secondary haemorrhage into the anterior chamber. This secondary haemorrhage may be a good deal more severe than the original one and is likely to cause secondary glaucoma. Such a secondary haemorrhage may occur within 10 days of the injury.

Most hyphaemas slowly absorb over about 7 days with rest. Full inspection of the retina through the dilated pupil is essential, once the hyphaema has cleared, to detect any associated retinal damage (Fig. 9.8).

Fig. 9.8
Hyphaema

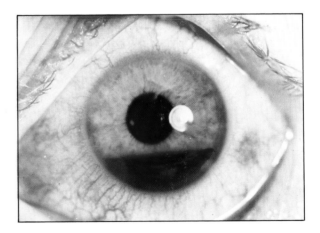

Iris disinsertion (iridodialysis)

The periphery of the iris is its weakest part and a concussion injury may cause tearing of the iris root giving an iridodialysis. The appearance is like an extra peripheral 'pupil'. An iridodialysis will be accompanied by a hyphaema at the time of the injury. Careful follow up of the patient will be essential because of the risk of secondary glaucoma later as a result of accompanying damage to the angle of the anterior chamber (Fig. 9.9).

Fig. 9.9
Iridodialysis

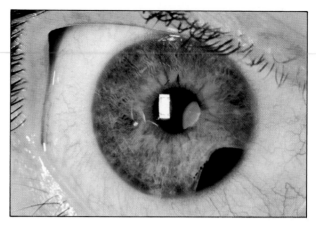

Lens subluxation

Any severe blow to the eye may cause displacement of the lens by rupturing the lens suspensory fibres. The lens may be displaced backwards in the vitreous (posterior subluxation or dislocation) or forwards into the anterior chamber (anterior subluxation or dislocation).

Lens subluxation requires long term specialist supervision because of the high risk of later secondary glaucoma and cataract formation. It can be recognised by the displacement of the lens in the pupil and by the tremulousness of the iris (iridodonesis) (Fig. 9.10).

Fig. 9.10
Subluxated lens

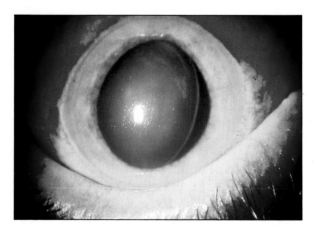

Intraocular foreign bodies

For a foreign body to penetrate the cornea or sclera and enter the eye it must be travelling at a very high velocity. Most are particles of metal and result from explosions, machinery, power tools and using a hammer and metal chisel. The patient normally experiences a foreign body sensation as the particle strikes the eye but occasionally it enters unnoticed. Sudden loss of vision and pain are also experienced as a rule.

Careful examination will reveal the small corneal or scleral wound at the point of entry and the foreign body itself in the iris or further back in the vitreous or retina. If the foreign body strikes the lens a cataract supervenes in a few hours. When an intraocular foreign body is suspected from the nature of the injury but none detected an X-ray of the ocular region will reveal a metallic foreign body (but not always a glass or plastic foreign body).

Treatment
Magnetic metallic foreign bodies may be removed at surgical operation with an electromagnet. Other intraocular foreign bodies such as lead or copper require removal using fine instruments manipulated within the eye (Fig. 9.11).

Fig. 9.11
Metal foreign body embedded in the iris

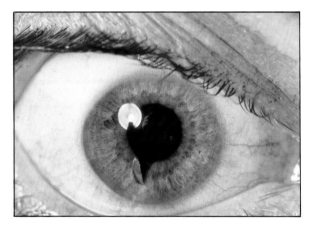

Penetrating injuries

Any sharp object may penetrate the eye to cause sudden loss of vision, pain, watering and redness of the eye. Examples include knives, screwdrivers, darts, flying metal and car windscreen glass.

Aqueous immediately leaks out of a corneal wound but the iris plugs or prolapses into the wound which forms the classical signs of a distorted pupil, shallowed anterior chamber and a visible external iris prolapse in a hyperaemic eye (Fig. 9.12).

Fig. 9.12
Perforating wound with prolapsed iris inferiorly

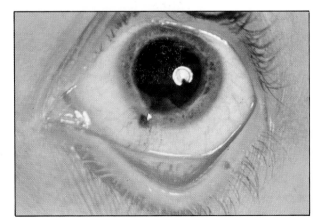

Treatment
Immediate surgical repair of the wound and replacement of the iris is necessary.

Retinal injuries and retinal detachment
A penetrating or concussion injury to the eye may cause retinal damage. Other visible signs of injury such as bruising of the eyelids, iridodialysis and subluxated lens should indicate the likelihood of accompanying retinal damage.

Retinal haemorrhage
Retinal haemorrhages following injury will be recognised with the ophthalmoscope providing there is no hyphaema preventing a clear view. The patient gives a history of injury and notices sudden loss of vision at the time of the injury. The retinal haemorrhages and oedema (Commotio retinae) are usually in the central area. No specific treatment is possible but slow resolution and some return of vision is likely over several weeks or months.

Choroidal ruptures
Splits in the choroid accompany severe concussion eye injuries with associated retinal haemorrhages and oedema. They may cause severe permanent visual impairment especially if a choroidal rupture underlies the central retina. The ophthalmoscopic appearance is that of whitish circumscribed streaks in the central fundus. The whitish appearance is because the choroidal ruptures allow the underlying sclera to be visualised (Fig. 9.13).

Fig. 9.13
Choroidal tears and haemorrhage

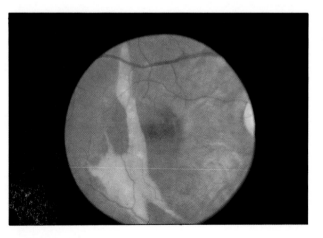

Retinal detachments
A retinal detachment is always associated with a break in the retina and any eye injury may cause this. With an injury the break is in the form of a retinal dialysis (or disinsertion) which appears as a well demarcated red area in the extreme periphery of the retina especially in the temporal area. A retinal detachment usually follows days or weeks after the injury.

If the retinal dialysis can be diagnosed before the detachment occurs, then the prognosis for vision is greatly improved. A retinal dialysis can be 'sealed off' by photocoagulation or cryotherapy, but once detachment has occurred then an extensive surgical operation is required (see Ch. 14).

Solar retinal burns

Looking directly at the sun may result in a burn of the central retina. This is especially common at the time of the sun's eclipse when many people inadvisably look directly at the sun.

There is rapid loss of vision as a result of central retinal oedema which is replaced over several weeks by fine macular scarring in the form of pigmentary clumping. No treatment is effective (Fig. 9.14).

Fig. 9.14
Solar macular burn

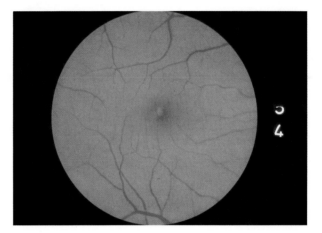

10

Strabismus (squint)

ANATOMY

Six extraocular muscles in each eye are responsible for eye movements (Fig. 10.1, 10.2). They are:

Superior rectus
Inferior rectus
Medial rectus   } Supplied by oculomotor nerve (III cranial nerve)
Inferior oblique

Superior oblique: Supplied by trochlear nerve (IV cranial nerve)
Lateral rectus: Supplied by abducent nerve (VI cranial nerve)

Before describing, defining and classifying the various types of squint it is necessary to describe the normal eye movements.

Visual axis

The visual axis is a useful descriptive term in discussing strabismus and normal eye movements. It is the theoretical line joining the point of fixation of the eye and the fovea of the retina. Eye movements are classified as follows:

Abduction, is the outward movement of the eye
Adduction, is the inward movement of the eye
Conjugate (or version) movements, when the eyes move together in parallel, i.e. looking to the left (laevoversion), looking to the right (dextroversion) or looking up, down and obliquely.
Disjunctive (or vergence) movements, when the eyes do not move together in parallel but their visual axes come together at a near point such as a book (convergence) or when in sleep or under sedation when the eyes deviate outwards symmetrically (divergence).

DEFINITION OF STRABISMUS

Strabismus or squint is present when the eyes do not conform to the normal parallelism or normal convergence and divergence and there are two main types:

Non-paralytic (concomitant) strabismus

This is the type of squint where the extraocular muscles are intact and the ocular movements are full in all directions of gaze. The angle of squint remains the same in all directions of gaze.

Fig. 10.1
Extraocular (extrinsic) muscles.
(Reproduced with kind permission of
the Hoya Corporation, Japan)

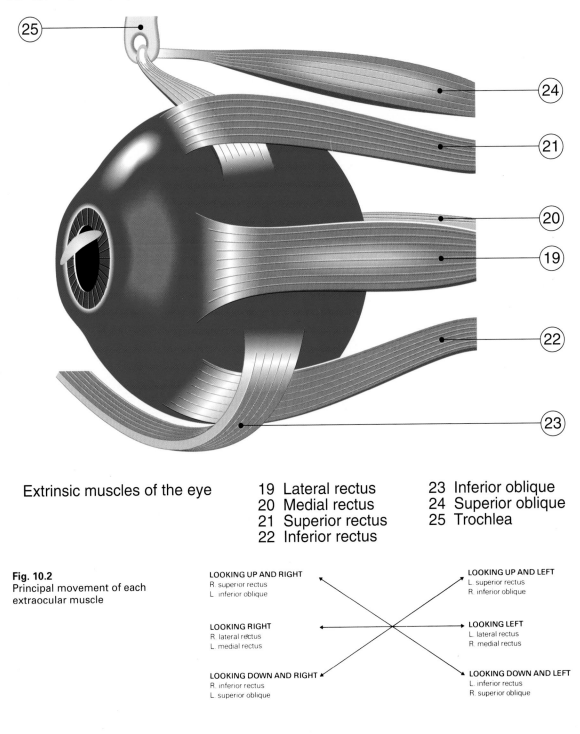

Extrinsic muscles of the eye

19	Lateral rectus	23	Inferior oblique
20	Medial rectus	24	Superior oblique
21	Superior rectus	25	Trochlea
22	Inferior rectus		

Fig. 10.2
Principal movement of each
extraocular muscle

LOOKING UP AND RIGHT
R. superior rectus
L. inferior oblique

LOOKING UP AND LEFT
L. superior rectus
R. inferior oblique

LOOKING RIGHT
R. lateral rectus
L. medial rectus

LOOKING LEFT
L. lateral rectus
R. medial rectus

LOOKING DOWN AND RIGHT
R. inferior rectus
L. superior oblique

LOOKING DOWN AND LEFT
L. inferior rectus
R. superior oblique

Paralytic (incomitant) strabismus
This is the type of squint caused by paralysis of one or more of the extraocular muscles or congenital abnormalities of the muscles. The angle of squint varies with the direction of gaze and the squint is at its maximum when looking in the direction of the action of the paralysed muscle.

NON-PARALYTIC (CONCOMITANT) STRABISMUS

The precise cause of a non-paralytic strabismus remains unknown except to say it is likely to be due to a failure within the brain to develop the complex binocular reflexes in early life. The frontal and occipital cortex of the cerebral hemispheres and the brain stem all influence ocular movement and its control. To an extent the development of these binocular reflexes can be influenced by the information the brain receives from the eyes so that high refractive errors or abnormalities of any structure within the eye may precipitate a squint. It is thus especially important to look for other associated abnormalities of the eyes before embarking on the definitive treatment of the strabismus.

Non-paralytic strabismus varies in its direction and is by far the most common type of squint occurring in children. The varieties of this condition are as follows:
1. Convergent squint (or esotropia), where the squinting eye turns inwards
2. Divergent squint (or exotropia), where the squinting eye turns outwards
3. Upward vertical squint (or hypertropia), where the squinting eye turns upwards
4. Downward vertical squint (or hypotropia), where the squinting eye turns downwards

Suppression and strabismic amblyopia
When strabismus occurs in infancy it seems likely that diplopia is present for a very short time only, if at all, and *suppression* of the unwanted image takes place by the visual cortex of the brain. Suppression may gradually become permanent so that the vision in the squinting eye is permanently severely reduced. This is *strabismic amblyopia*. If strabismus occurs from birth or in the first few months of life then the normal vision in the squinting eye never develops and this type of amblyopia is *amblyopia of arrest*. When vision develops normally, say, for the first two or three years of life and a squint occurs then suppression and *amblyopia of suppression* will occur in the squinting eye.

Suppression $\longrightarrow$ Strabismic amblyopia $\begin{cases} \text{Amblyopia of arrest} \\ \\ \text{Suppression amblyopia} \end{cases}$

Importance of early diagnosis

The importance of early diagnosis of childhood strabismus is threefold:

1. To exclude an abnormality of the squinting eye, e.g. cataract or retinoblastoma
2. To reverse the effects of suppression and prevent amblyopia of the squinting eye
3. To straighten the eye to alleviate parental anxiety and avoid any social or educational disadvantage for the child

Presenting features of strabismus

Undoubtedly the majority of infants present because they are noticed to have eyes which are not in alignment but occasionally the squint is only detected at a routine vision test, say at school, when the amblyopia is noted. This applies to small angle squints in particular. There is a familial tendency for squint to occur so parents may ask for an infant to be examined because of this. Hence the presenting features in strabismus are:

1. Misalignment of the eyes (convergent, divergent etc.)
2. Poor vision in one eye detected at routine examination
3. Family history of squint.

Age of onset

Most concomitant strabismus in infants has its onset between the ages of 1 and 3 years. However a proportion of squints are congenital.

Clinical features of strabismus

History: A careful history from the parents of the infant should elicit the following features:

1. Age of onset
2. Direction of the strabismus, i.e. whether convergent, divergent etc.
3. The variability of the squint or whether it is constant
4. The details of *birth history* such as birth weight and any perinatal events (strabismus is more common in cerebral palsy for example)
5. Any family history of strabismus

Examination procedure

The following methods should be employed in the examination for strabismus:

Face inspection, looking especially for abnormalities of the skull and orbits.

Ocular movements, an infant will follow a bright pen torch light and the range of movement of the eyes can be estimated.

Visual acuity, measurement in each eye separately. In infants this can best be estimated by eliciting optico-kinetic nystagmus. Children of about 3 years and over will usually perform the Sheridan-Gardiner test of matching letters (see Ch. 1).

Fig. 10.3
Corneal reflections observed in a child with a convergent squint

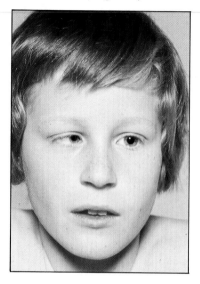

The angle of the strabismus, and its direction can be estimated using a bright pen torch light and observing the *corneal reflections* of this light. The light is held about 50 cm *in the mid line* in front of the infant's face. If the reflected light image from each cornea is asymmetrical then a squint is present (Fig. 10.3, 10.4).

The cover test: The child is asked to look at a fixation object held about one metre in front of the face, or in the case of infants a bright pen torch light may be used. Each eye in turn is then covered by an occluder or the examiner's hand. If the uncovered eye then moves to take up fixation a squint is present. The direction of squint is given by the opposite of the direction in which the eye moves, i.e. convergent, divergent etc. When the cover is removed the squinting eye may continue fixing until it is again covered. This is an alternating squint and indicates equal vision in each eye (Fig. 10.5).

Full examination of the eyes, including ophthalmoscopy and refraction by retinoscopy after instillation of cycloplegic eye drops (Cyclopentolate or Tropicamide 1%).

In specialist ophthalmic departments further evaluation of the state of the binocular vision and more precise methods of measuring the angle of squint are employed in older children. These methods include the use of the prism bar cover test, the foveoscope and the synoptophore.

Treatment of strabismus: The majority of squints in infants and children are convergent (or esotropia), being about four times more common than the divergent squint (or exotropia). Treatment is directed towards achieving the best possible vision, reversing suppression and amblyopia if possible and improving binocular vision with straightening of the eyes (Fig. 10.3, 10.4).

Refractive errors, when significant are corrected with spectacles (or contact lenses in older children especially where there is a high refractive error). Many children with convergent strabismus have hypermetropic refractive errors. Any spectacles prescribed should be in duplicate, to cater for repairs, and have plastic or toughened glass lenses. Even infants of 12 months of age may tolerate spectacles.

Fig. 10.4
Divergent strabismus. (Courtesy of the Western Ophthalmic Hospital)

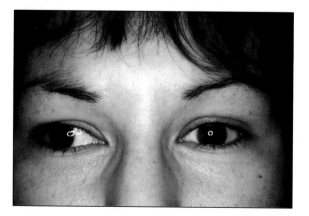

Fig. 10.5
The cover test

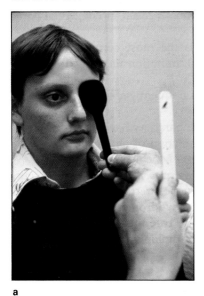

a

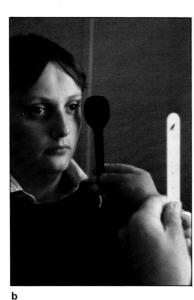

b

Occlusion: This method is used in an attempt to reverse suppression and amblyopia. An adhesive patch or occluder is worn over the 'good' or non-squinting eye for 4–6 weeks initially *providing improvement in the vision in the squinting eye is occurring*. If the strabismus is long standing, with amblyopia, the occlusion treatment may fail to improve the vision and this is especially so after the age of 6 years. Sometimes a child will not tolerate the occluder and in this situation Atropine ½% eye drops may be instilled into the 'good' eye in order to blur the vision and encourage fixation in the squinting eye.

Orthoptic exercises, are only applicable for older children as clearly an infant will be unable to cooperate with the synoptophore, for example. The principle of orthoptic exercises is to overcome suppression and encourage fusion of the two images by stimulating both retinal foveas simultaneously with picture images presented to the child in a synoptophore machine. Other methods used involve bar reading, which can be done as a home exercise, and stimulating the fovea of an amblyopic eye with a rotating striped disc.

Surgical operation: The principle of surgical treatment of strabismus is to align the two visual axes. This is achieved by shortening (strengthening) one muscle and lengthening (weakening) its fellow muscle by adjusting the muscle insertions on the sclera. For most squints this involves the medial and lateral rectus muscles in one eye (uniocular operation), twin operations on both medial or both lateral recti muscles (binocular operation) and sometimes additional adjustment of the superior and inferior oblique muscles.

For example, a convergent strabismus will require lengthening (*a recession*) of the medial rectus muscle and shortening (*a resection*) of the lateral rectus muscle; alternatively the medial rectus muscle in each eye may be recessed.

The precise choice of surgical operation and the amount of lengthening and shortening required depends on the type of squint, the angle of squint and the extent of binocular vision.

When full restoration of binocular function is achieved after surgery then the operation is *curative*. If irreversible amblyopia is present the operation may be undertaken to achieve an improved *cosmetic* appearance.

PARALYTIC (INCOMITANT) STRABISMUS

Paralytic strabismus is the result of interruption of the motor nerve pathway to one or more of the extraocular muscles. Complete loss of muscle function is a *paralysis* whereas partial loss is a *paresis*.

Paralytic strabismus is readily detected because of the presence of the squint and the *limitation of eye movement* in the direction of action of the affected muscle.

The majority of paralytic squints are acquired in later life as a result of systemic disease, although there are some which are *congenital*.

Meningitis and encephalomyelitis
Multiple cranial nerve paralyses may occur in these conditions caused by many different bacteria and viruses.

Multiple sclerosis
This condition affecting the whole nervous system and occurring in young people may cause III, IV and VI cranial nerve paralyses.

Intracranial neoplasms and aneurysms
III, IV and VI cranial nerve paralysis frequently accompany cerebral, cerebellar and mid-brain neoplasms. In fact the squint and diplopia may be the first clinical sign of such an intracranial neoplasm. Sudden onset of cranial nerve paralyses may also be due to cerebral aneurysms (usually on the circle of Willis).

Myasthenia gravis
Generalised muscle weakness occurs in patients due to failure of neuromuscular junctions to adequately transmit impulses. Diplopia due to extraocular muscle paralysis and ptosis, are frequent presenting features which characteristically vary in their severity being worse with tiredness.

Thyrotoxicosis
Individual extraocular muscle weakness, especially of the superior rectus muscles, gives rise to diplopia and often accompanies thyrotoxicosis.

Treatment of paralytic strabismus
This initially involves treatment of the underlying cause after which any remaining paralytic squint may be treated definitively following an interval of at least 6 months as some spontaneous recovery may take place during this period.

Prism spectacles may assist the diplopia in small angle paralytic squints but frequently surgical operation is required to correct the diplopia and abnormal head posture. The principle of surgical treatment is to shorten (weaken) the over acting paired (synergist) muscle in the other eye. This is because surgical operations directly on the paralysed muscle (shortening or resection operations) are not very successful.

Botulinum neurotoxin A also has a use in treatment of paralytic squint, e.g. VIth nerve palsy. The ocular muscle is injected under local anaesthetic with the toxin. Botulinum neurotoxin A acts by preventing acetycholine release at the synaptic nerve terminal.

11

Cataract and lens displacement

ANATOMY AND DEVELOPMENT

The crystalline lens develops from ectoderm by invaginating into the primitive optic vesicle. This accounts for the close relationship between many ectodermal (mainly skin) conditions and cataract. Two skin conditions associated with cataract are atopic eczema and scleroderma. The ciliary zonule made up of fine suspensory fibres holds the lens in position but allows it to alter its surface curvature and thickness (*accommodation*) to focus images clearly on the retina.

Clinical slit lamp microscope examination of the lens reveals the characteristic transparent structure but various layers can be identified giving a clear observation of the laying down of the lens fibres from the embryo to birth. The lens fibres are laid down from the epithelial layer lying at the most anterior portion of the lens and arranged in such a precise and regular way that the lens is characteristically transparent (Fig. 11.1, 11.2).

Fig. 11.1
The lens in position in the anterior part of the eye

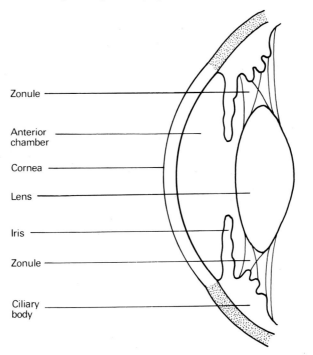

Zonule

Anterior chamber

Cornea

Lens

Iris

Zonule

Ciliary body

Fig. 11.2
Section through a lens

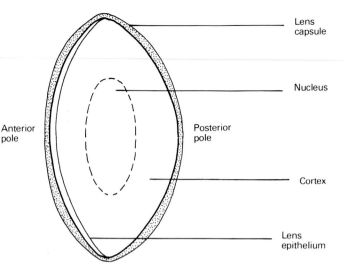

Lens capsule

Nucleus

Anterior pole

Posterior pole

Cortex

Lens epithelium

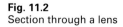

CATARACT

A cataract is any opacity of the crystalline lens, some of which are such minor variations in transparency that they do not affect vision. Types of cataract are classified as follows
1. Developmental cataracts
2. Congenital cataracts
3. Senile cataracts
4. Cataracts secondary to ocular disease
5. Cataracts associated with systemic disease

DEVELOPMENTAL CATARACTS

These are minor opacities in the transparency of the lens and do not affect vision but are worthy of note in order to recognise that they are harmless when observed in patients being examined for other reasons. There are three types of developmental cataract which can be observed in a high proportion of the normal population and may be present at birth or develop in the first few years of life. It should be stressed that all three types (described below) are harmless:

Coronary lens opacities
These are whitish or bluish finger shape opacities in the periphery of the lens cortex. They can usually only be seen with the pupil dilated.

Blue dot lens opacities

Whitish or bluish dot opacities of varying size occur in the cortex of the lens in many people in the normal population (Fig. 11.3).

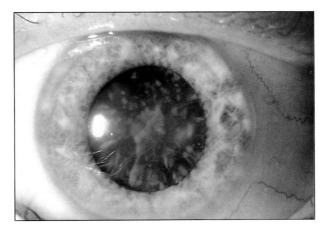

Fig. 11.3
Blue dot and coronary developmental lens opacities; a more marked example than usual

Dilacerated lens opacities

This type of lens opacity is relatively unusual but appears as a striking bluish, fern leaf-like opacity in the lens cortex.

CONGENITAL CATARACTS

Congenital cataracts are usually bilateral but unilateral ones may also occur. Probably in the majority of infants the cause is not known, however, they may be familial, either as the result of intra-uterine infection (especially rubella), or drugs taken during pregnancy or they may be associated with other congenital defects such as syphilis, galactosaemia, diabetes mellitus and Down's syndrome.

Symptoms
1. The appearance of a white or grey pupil(s)
2. A manifest strabismus (squint)
3. Nystagmus

Nystagmus is an indication of severe visual impairment and may vary from fine pendular nystagmus to wide ranging irregular movements. With unilateral cataract in particular, another associated cause should be looked for, e.g. retinoblastoma, toxoplasmosis and the presence of microphthalmos.

Types of congenital cataract

Lamellar (Zonular) cataract

This type of cataract derives its name because it occupies a zone or layer within the lens nucleus. About 40% of all congenital cataracts are Lamellar (Fig. 11.4).

Fig. 11.4
Lamellar cataract: note clear periphery of lens

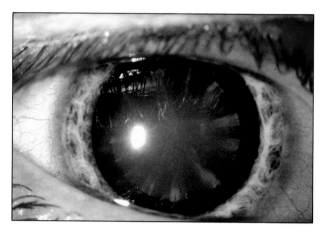

Anterior and posterior polar cataracts

These lens opacities are confined to the anterior or posterior poles of the lens respectively. Usually they are small and affect vision to a degree in proportion to their size. They are often associated with fibrous vascular remnants such as a persistent hyaloid artery in the vitreous (Fig. 11.5).

Fig. 11.5
Posterior polar congenital cataract

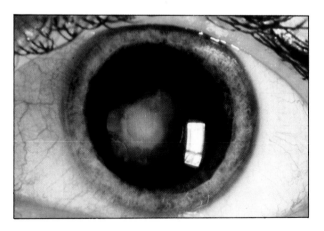

Nuclear cataract

As well as the more common zonular cataract other varying forms of nuclear cataract occur. These may be simple powder-like white spots in the nucleus of the lens (pulverulent cataract) or total opacification of the nucleus.

Fig. 11.6
'Lensectomy' for congenital cataract

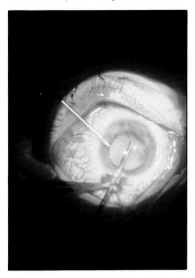

Treatment

Where the cataract is not interfering significantly with the infant's general development and the vision can be assessed as reasonable then no treatment is required. When the infant's vision is severely impaired, as when nystagmus is present, then surgery is required to remove the cataract. For cataracts in the central portion of the lens only, e.g. lamellar or polar cataracts, mydriatic eye drops may be used to keep the pupils dilated which allows adequate vision through the clear lens periphery.

When surgery is required the methods of choice for congenital cataracts are 'lensectomy' (phaco-fragmentation), lens aspiration or lens discission (Fig. 11.6).

After operation contact lenses may be fitted in most infants or alternatively spectacles at a suitable age.

SENILE CATARACT

This type of cataract refers to the primary age-associated lens opacities. Senile or senescent cataracts form the great majority of all cataracts and can be widely observed in the general population. Almost all people over the age of 65 years have some degree of cataract. They may occur earlier in life (sometimes called pre-senile cataracts) especially in people where nutrition has been poor or who have diabetes mellitus. It is important to distinguish three types of senile cataract because each type has a different outlook and speed of development. In general, however, the symptoms of all types of senile cataract are similar.

Symptoms

1. Slowly progressive, painless decrease in visual acuity. This may take place over several months or years and usually affects both eyes
2. Glare in bright lights and sunlight
3. Fixed, dark 'spots' in the field of vision
4. Poor colour vision
5. Double or multiple images seen with one eye (polyopia)

Types of senile cataract

Nuclear sclerosis

This is a very slow, progressive, yellowing and hardening of the lens nucleus. In this way the refractive index of the lens is increased and this renders the patient more myopic. Such patients continue to see small print and may even be able to abandon their spectacles for reading. This often gives rise to bemused comments by relatives such as, 'isn't granny wonderful reading without spectacles at her age—'. Hence with this type of cataract it is safe to indicate to the patient that he will be able to manage to see small print for many years to come even if the distance vision does become progressively blurred (Fig. 11.7).

Fig. 11.7
Nuclear sclerosis

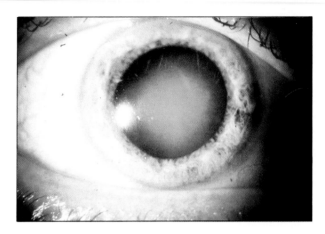

Cuneiform cataract

These are radially arranged spoke-like opacities appearing at the lens periphery both in the anterior and the posterior cortex which slowly extend to the central area of the lens thereby affecting vision. Cuneiform opacities progress very slowly over many years and patients may be reassured that their progressive visual deterioration will be correspondingly slow (Fig. 11.8).

Fig. 11.8
Cuneiform cataract by (a) direct
illumination and (b) seen against red
fundus reflex

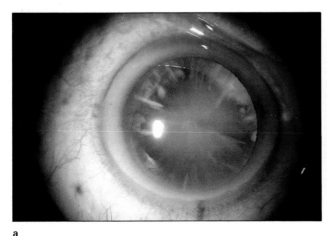

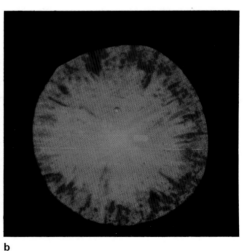

a   b

Posterior subcapsular (cupuliform) cataract

This is another form of cortical cataract but unlike the other two types of senile cataract the opacities progress fairly rapidly. The opacities commence in the central (axial) portion of the lens immediately beneath the posterior lens capsule and extend peripherally. Because of their axial position, close to the theoretical nodal point of the reduced eye, they may have a rapid and profound effect on vision. Hence the need to warn patients with this type of cataract that they may need treatment relatively soon (Fig. 11.9).

Fig. 11.9
Posterior subcapsular cataract in (a) direct illumination and (b) against the red fundus reflex

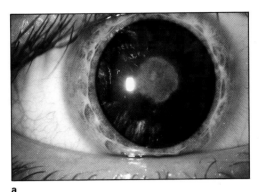

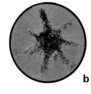

a

Nuclear sclerosis, cuneiform and cupuliform opacities may also occur together or in combinations of two types. Nuclear sclerosis occurs particularly in myopic patients and cupuliform opacities are also associated with patients having systemic steroid treatment.

When a senile cataract occupies the whole lens it is often called a *mature cataract* and in these circumstances there is no view of the red fundus reflex with the ophthalmoscope (Fig. 11.10).

Fig. 11.10
Mature or complete cataract

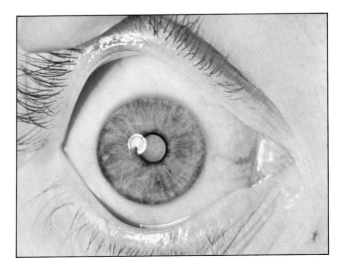

Evaluation of senile cataract

1. Estimation of corrected visual acuity with spectacles.
2. Examination for other disease especially glaucoma and retinal disease. Macular degeneration in particular should be carefully sought for as this will greatly affect the timing of the cataract operation.
3. Documentation of the type of cataract as this usually influences the prognosis.
4. The patient's occupation, general health, interests and hobbies should be recorded in order to assess an individual patient's visual needs.
5. Where a unilateral senile cataract occurs in particular it is important to seek other causes such as previous trauma, uveitis and intraocular foreign body.

Extracapsular cataract extraction and posterior chamber intraocular lens implantation is now the standard technique for cataract treatment. The technique refers to removing the lens substance (nucleus and cortex) piecemeal and leaving the posterior lens capsule intact. Most patients now have this operation performed as a day operation under local or general anaesthetic. The suitability of the patient for local anaesthetic is determined by factors such as the patient's general health, age and the personal wishes of the patient and the preference of the operating surgeon. The operating microscope is used. An incision is made in the peripheral corneal margin superiorly and a central disc of anterior capsule removed or alternatively a linear opening in the capsule formed. The nucleus of the lens is then gently expressed from the eye through the opening in the capsule and through the corneal incision. The remaining lens cortex is then removed piecemeal by irrigation and aspiration through a mechanised handpiece. Instead of the separate lens nucleus expression, with irrigation and aspiration of the lens cortex, the *phacoemulsification* technique is widely used. This consists of removing the lens nucleus and cortex by ultrasonic vibrations before aspiration with the handpiece (Fig. 11.11).

Once the lens nucleus and cortex have been removed a *posterior chamber intraocular lens implant* is placed into the capsular bag. Fine sutures unite the corneal incision and full mobilisation of the patient occurs at once.

Intracapsular cataract extraction is a technique now seldom used. This operation requires the removal of the lens intact with its capsule by forceps or cryoprobe through a corneal incision. The technique is outdated because it makes the insertion of a capsule supported posterior chamber lens implant unsuitable. An anterior chamber lens implant may be used with the intracapsular technique but this carries a higher complication rate such as secondary glaucoma and corneal oedema.

Aphakic vision and intraocular lens implants

Removing a cataractous lens in a patient results in aphakia (absence of the lens). The aphakic eye has lost its power of accommodation

Fig. 11.11
General operation view showing operating microscope

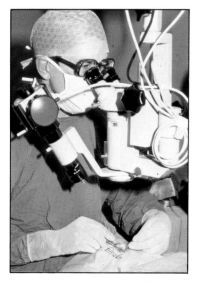

and is on average rendered 10 dioptres hypermetropic (long sighted). Hence, in order to see clearly a patient requires the equivalent high powered convex spectacles, a contact lens or now routinely used, an *intraocular lens implant*.

Spectacles to correct aphakia do have the disadvantage of making the patient entirely dependent on them and require many months of adaptation to the 25% magnified image and peripheral distortion of the spectacle lenses. Judgement of distances especially when pouring liquids and descending steps is a particular problem. These major disadvantages of removing a cataractous lens without an intraocular lens implant led to the now routine use of the *posterior chamber intraocular lens implant*.

A *contact lens* fitted after operation overcomes the high magnification and distortion of spectacles. However, many elderly patients have difficulty in handling a contact lens and regular follow-up examinations may be required. Hence a contact lens has been replaced by the intraocular lens implant.

Intraocular lens implants (lens implants) are routinely used as they overcome the disadvantages of spectacles and contact lenses. These implants are made of polymethylmethacrylate and are inserted into the eye at the time of cataract extraction. The routinely used lens implant is the *posterior chamber implant* (Fig. 11.12) which is situated exactly in the anatomical position of the original crystalline lens. An extracapsular cataract removal technique is essential for this lens implant to maintain its position.

Fig. 11.12
Posterior chamber lens implant: note lower margin of implant not normally easily seen because it lies behind the iris

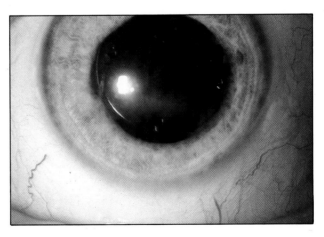

Folding posterior chamber lens implants are increasingly being used and have the obvious advantage of allowing a smaller corneal incision through which to introduce the folding lens implant. Once the folding lens is introduced through the small incision it opens up in the capsular bag.

An *anterior chamber implant* is occasionally used and either an intracapsular or extracapsular cataract removal technique may be used. The anterior chamber lens implant is held in position by the attached supports in the angle of the anterior chamber (Fig. 11.13). Anterior chamber lens implants are only now used for previously aphakic patients for secondary implantation.

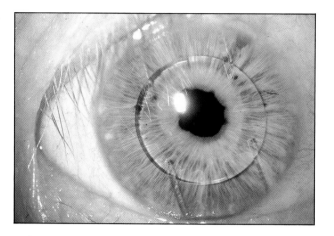

Fig. 11.13
Anterior chamber lens implant: note supporting limbs above and below

CATARACTS SECONDARY TO OCULAR DISEASE

Many ocular conditions can cause cataracts, the main ones being:
1. Iritis
2. Injury (both penetrating and non-penetrating injuries) and radiation
3. Keratitis
4. Neovascular (haemorrhagic or thrombotic glaucoma)

CATARACTS ASSOCIATED WITH SYSTEMIC DISEASE

A large number of congenital and systemic disorders are associated with cataracts. Some of them are described below:

Systemic disorders

Diabetes mellitus
The cataracts in diabetes are the same as senile cataracts except they occur a decade or so earlier in diabetics of long standing and progress more rapidly.

Hypoparathyroidism
Fine, white, flake-like opacities in the lens cortex, only minimally affecting vision, occur in hypoparathyroidism. The site of the opacities in the cortex correspond in all probability to the periods of hypocalcaemia.

Dystrophia myotonica

This hereditary disease, characterised by frontal baldness, generalised muscle wasting giving an expressionless face, and testicular atrophy, is associated with fine, white, dot cataracts sited in the lens cortex.

Systemic steroid treatment

Patients receiving high dose systemic steroid therapy for various conditions over long periods may develop characteristic posterior subcapsular cataracts as a complication.

Congenital disorders

Down's syndrome

A number of different cataracts occur in this condition which results from a chromosome defect (chromosome 21 Trisomy). However, most of these types do not seriously impair vision and seldom require treatment.

Galactosaemia

Cataracts are a frequent feature of this inherited disorder of carbohydrate metabolism.

DISPLACEMENT OF THE LENS (ECTOPIA LENTIS)

Complete displacement (dislocation) or partial displacement (subluxation) of the lens may be congenital or acquired. When congenital it is usually symmetrically bilateral and may occur as an isolated anomaly or can be part of a general spread of systemic abnormalities. Defective suspensory fibres of the zonule holding the lens in place account for this displacement.

Features of a displaced lens

1. Tremulousness or 'wobbling' of the iris is apparent (iridodenesis) owing to the iris no longer being supported by the lens. Iridodenesis is also a constant feature observed in the eye following cataract extraction.
2. Through the dilated pupil the fundus may be observed partly through the lens and partly past the edge of the lens (Fig. 11.14).
3. The edge of the displaced lens can often be observed in the pupil.
4. If the lens is displaced into the anterior chamber (anterior dislocation) secondary glaucoma may occur rapidly owing to interruption of normal aqueous outflow by the lens from the angle. In such circumstances the pupil should be dilated and the patient laid flat on his back in an attempt to allow the lens to fall back behind the iris. If this is successful then the pupil should be immediately constricted with miotic drops. If unsuccessful, operation to remove the lens must be performed at once. When

Fig. 11.14
Lens subluxation

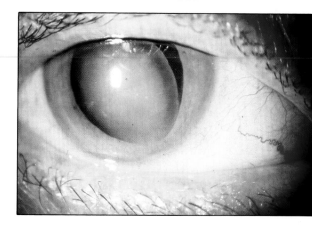

the lens is displaced posteriorly into the vitreous (posterior sub-luxation) further possible complications are cataract, uveitis and secondary glaucoma.

5. Rapid changes in the patient's vision associated with rapid changes in refractive error frequently occur with subluxated lenses because of the mobility of the lens. Increasing myopia occurs as the lens moves posteriorly and when the lens is displaced away from the central pupil area the eye is effectively rendered 'aphakic' thereby requiring appropriate spectacles or contact lenses.

Conditions associated with subluxated lenses

Marfan's syndrome
Long fingers and toes (arachnodactyly), tall stature, high arched palate, congenital heart defects and subluxated lenses.

Homocystinuria
A metabolic disorder of infants characterised by mental retardation, fair complexion and hair, spastic gait, chest wall deformities and subluxated lenses.

Injuries
Concussion or penetrating injuries to the eye may cause rupture of part of the len's suspensory fibres with consequent lens displacement.

Senility
Spontaneous rupture of the lens suspensory fibres may occur in older people especially associated with advanced cataract and myopia.

12

Glaucoma

The word glaucoma is derived from the Greek 'glaucos' meaning green, possibly as a result of an erroneous observation of cataracts in Ancient Greece.

Definition
Glaucoma is a condition affecting usually both eyes in which there is visual field loss, raised intraocular pressure and excavation or pathological cupping of the optic disc. The raised intraocular pressure causes ischaemia of the optic nerve head with consequent damage to retinal nerve fibres resulting in loss of visual field.

Incidence
Glaucoma is a common condition in the population and affects some 1.5% of people over 40. There is a familial incidence, thus affected patients should alert close relatives of the possibility of undiagnosed glaucoma, especially in siblings. It is one of the world's most common causes of blindness.

ANATOMY AND PHYSIOLOGY

The angle of the anterior chamber which features in the classification of glaucoma refers to the anatomical angle between the cornea and the iris. Contained in the angle is the trabecular meshwork, a series of interweaved fibres communicating with the canal of Schlemm (modified vein). Aqueous, secreted from the ciliary body, passes through the pupil into the anterior chamber angle and thence through the trabecular meshwork spaces into the canal of Schlemm (Fig. 12.1, 12.2).

This constant production, flow and exit of aqueous within the eye maintains a more or less constant intraocular pressure within the range 11–22 mmHg. When the outflow of aqueous is embarrassed a rise of intraocular pressure occurs and glaucoma supervenes. In the case of acute glaucoma the obstruction occurs at the periphery of the iris and pressure rises in a few hours. In chronic glaucoma the site of obstruction is the trabecular meshwork and in this case pressure rises over months and even years, so that damage to the optic nerve head (disc) with subsequent loss of the field of vision is gradual.

Fig. 12.1
Anterior segment of the eye

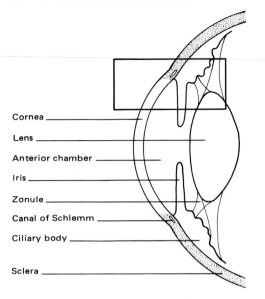

Cornea

Lens

Anterior chamber

Iris

Zonule

Canal of Schlemm

Ciliary body

Sclera

Fig. 12.2
The angle of the anterior chamber

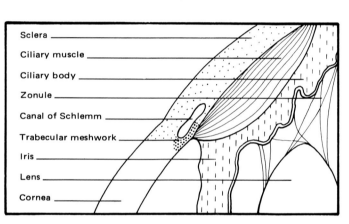

Sclera

Ciliary muscle

Ciliary body

Zonule

Canal of Schlemm

Trabecular meshwork

Iris

Lens

Cornea

Fig. 12.3
The gonioscope

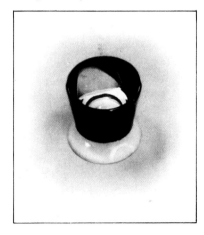

The angle of the anterior chamber is visualised clinically on the slit lamp microscope using a modified contact lens (a gonioscope) placed on the anaesthetised cornea (Fig. 12.3, 12.4, 12.5).

CLASSIFICATION OF GLAUCOMA

Primary glaucomas are those not associated with other ocular conditions while secondary glaucomas are those which occur as a result of other ocular or systemic diseases.

Fig. 12.4
The principle of gonioscopy

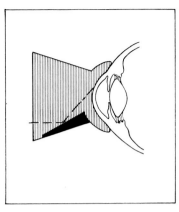

Fig. 12.5
Gonioscope view of normal open angle

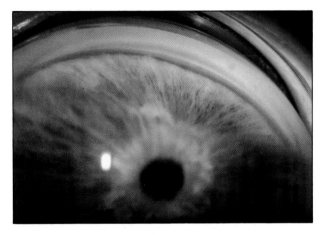

PRIMARY GLAUCOMAS

This group is the most common and will be encountered in all aspects of ophthalmic practice. The recognition of primary glaucomas in the early stages is fundamental to prevention of blindness. The group may be classified as follows:

1. Chronic simple (open angle) glaucoma
2. Acute (closed angle) glaucoma
3. Congenital glaucoma (buphthalmos)

Chronic simple (open angle) glaucoma

Because of the gradual rise of intraocular pressure in chronic simple glaucoma the symptoms may be very gradual and the condition frequently goes unnoticed in the early stages. The condition is usually bilateral and affects the over 40s but is most common after the age of 60 years. Approximately 1–2% of the over 40s are affected, hence it is one of the most common worldwide blinding diseases. Chronic open angle glaucoma is frequently inherited and some 10% of first degree relatives of affected individuals also eventually develop glaucoma. Hence it is desirable that first degree relatives of glaucoma sufferers should receive regular routine examinations after the age of 40 years.

Symptoms
1. Loss of part of the visual field. This may be noticed by the patient as 'bumping into things'
2. Gradual deterioration of close vision. This is more rapid than the usual presbyopic failure of accommodation in the over 40s and the patient may ascribe this failure in vision to the need for stronger reading spectacles
3. Routine medical and optometric examinations frequently detect glaucoma from the appearance of the optic discs or the detection of visual field loss. No opportunity should ever be allowed to pass to examine the optic discs of patients attending for medical examinations for any purpose. By this means screening of the population for glaucoma may be achieved.

Signs
1. The optic disc is pathologically cupped (excavated) and pale with the central retinal vessels displaced nasally on the disc surface. Evaluation of the size of the cup is helped by observing the cup in relation to the disc (cup/disc or C/D ratio) in the vertical meridian (Fig. 12.6). A disc with a C/D ratio of 0.5 or less is unlikely to be glaucomatous. Greater than 0.5, however, is increasingly likely to be glaucomatous (Fig. 12.7).

   The paleness or pallor of the disc is estimated from how much area of the disc lacks small blood vessels; this area of the disc which is pale is constant in the normal disc but increases in glaucoma (and other causes of optic atrophy). Hence in chronic open angle glaucoma the area of cupping and pallor of the disc progressively increase together.

Fig. 12.6
The cup/disc ratio

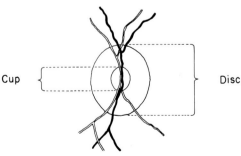

Cup

Disc

Fig. 12.7
A glaucomatous disc showing
excavation (pathological cupping)
and atrophy with a C/D ratio 0.8

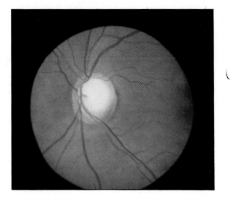

2. Visual field defects occur which can be plotted by perimetry
   and they are, characteristically, the arcuate scotoma, an enlarged
   blind spot and the nasal step defect (Fig. 12.8).

Fig. 12.8
Field defects in chronic glaucoma

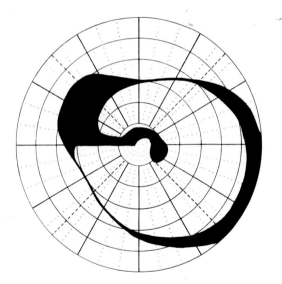

3. Raised intraocular pressure usually in the range 28–40 mmHg
   measured by tonometry. Tonometry may only be satisfactorily
   performed by the specialist using the slit lamp microscope
   applanation tonometer.

   It should be emphasised that these signs are all 'internal' to the
   eye and there are no apparent external signs. This is in marked
   contrast to acute glaucoma where all the signs are external.

Treatment

Chronic simple glaucoma is controlled using medical treatment initially and operation is usually reserved for those patients in which this fails to control the loss of the field of vision. Treatment consists of the use of one or more type of eye drop instilled daily although the frequency and strength of the drops used vary from patient to patient.

Medical treatments used in chronic glaucoma are as follows (used separately or in combinations):

1. *Beta-adrenergic blockade eye drops*
   Timolol maleate 0.25–0.5% (Timoptol, Timolol, Timoptic), betaxolol (Betoptic), carteolol (Teoptic), metipranolol (Glauline), levobunolol (Betagan).
   Instil twice daily.
   Action: lowers ocular pressure by reducing aqueous humour formation.

2. *Parasympathomimetic eye drops*
   Pilocarpine 1–6%
   Eserine 0.25–0.5%
   Carbachol 0.75–3%
   Instil two to four times daily.
   Action: increases facility of outflow of aqueous probably by the mechanical effect via ciliary muscle contraction pulling on the opening of the trabecular meshwork.

3. *Sympathomimetic eye drops*
   Neutral adrenaline 0.5–1% (Simplene, Eppy, Epifrin)
   Instil twice daily.
   Action: decreases aqueous humour formation.

4. *Adrenergic blockade eye drops*
   Guanethidine monosulphate 5% (Ismelin)
   Guanethidine combined with neutral adrenaline, varying combinations (Ganda)
   Instil twice daily.
   Action of guanethidine: potentiates adrenaline.

5. *Carbonic anhydrase inhibitor*
   Acetazolamide (Diamox) tablets or parenteral preparation 250 mg–1 g in divided doses by mouth. (Intravenous use is particularly applicable in acute angle closure glaucoma – see pages 89–91).
   Action: decreases aqueous humour production by inhibiting carbonic anhydrase in the ciliary body.

Once a diagnosis of chronic open angle glaucoma has been made treatment commences with twice daily beta-adrenergic blockade eye drops (typically Timolol). The patient is monitored every few weeks until the intraocular pressures fall to a normal level. Should the initial treatment be insufficient then typically *additional* parasympathomimetic eye drops are added (pilocarpine) or sympathomimetic drops (adrenaline) or adrenergic blockade drops (guanethidine). In most patients the initial treatment of beta-adrenergic blockade drops is sufficient to control the intraocular pressure and prevent further visual field loss. Additional medication as above is required should control not be adequate.

Side effects of beta-adrenergic eye drops are uncommon but include bradycardia and dyspnoea due to bronchospasm. Pilocarpine has the major side effect of pupil constriction (miosis) which blurs vision and reduces night vision especially. Much reduced side effects are achieved with Pilocarpine wafer inserts (Ocusert Pilo) which are placed under the upper eyelid and slowly release Pilocarpine (Fig. 12.9). They are changed weekly. Sympathomimetic eye drops (adrenaline) may cause conjunctival vessel dilatation (injection), palpitations and tachycardia. A carbonic anhydrase inhibitor (Diamox) is generally used for short periods, say, during the initial controlling period after diagnosis or whilst waiting for laser or surgical treatment. Diamox side effects may be serious and are malaise, diarrhoea, anorexia, paraesthesiae, kidney stones and blood dyscrasias. Hence Diamox is used intravenously largely in acute angle closure glaucoma and for short periods whilst achieving control of open angle glaucoma.

Fig. 12.9
Ocusert in position on its way under upper eyelid

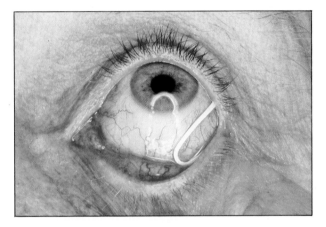

Surgical treatment in chronic glaucoma may be required when medical treatment fails to control the progressive loss of the visual field and raised intraocular pressure. The operation most used is *trabeculectomy* in which a surgical fistula is fashioned from the anterior chamber angle allowing aqueous to leave the eye by this alternative channel. *Laser trabeculoplasty* is a technique which may be performed as an out-patient procedure and consists of placing argon laser burns to form small spaces in the trabecular meshwork and hence improve aqueous drainage. It is less effective than surgical operation in reducing intraocular pressure but indicated in cases of moderate glaucoma.

Acute (closed angle) glaucoma

Acute glaucoma develops rapidly over several hours hence producing striking and obvious external eye signs. There is an anatomical predisposition in these patients by virtue of narrow anterior chamber

Fig. 12.10
Acute glaucoma

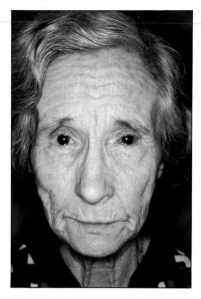

angles, but usually only one eye at a time is affected. The onset is often in the evening and precipitated by emotional or physical upset in the over 40s age group with a peak incidence around 60–70 years of age.

Symptoms

1. Rapid loss of vision over several hours (due to the corneal oedema)
2. Pain in the region of the eye and orbit which is severe and aching in character and may give rise to nausea
3. The eye is red, watery and photophobic
4. Haloes (rainbow coloured rings) may be seen round small artificial light sources and this symptom may precede the acute attack on occasions days or weeks beforehand. This effect is caused by diffraction in the oedematous cornea

Signs

1. The eye is red due to dilatation of the ciliary vessels especially noticeable round the corneal margin, the limbus, giving rise to the circumcorneal or ciliary hyperaemia
2. The cornea is cloudy due to corneal oedema
3. The pupil is half dilated, oval and unreacting to pupil reflexes
4. There is a very high intraocular pressure in the region of 60–70 mmHg easily detected by digital palpation with the index fingers (Fig. 12.10, 12.11)

Fig. 12.11
The eye signs in acute glaucoma

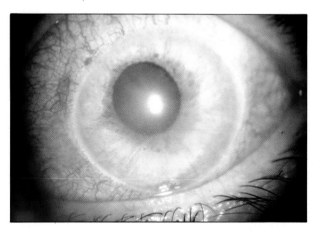

Treatment

Acute glaucoma is a medical emergency. Delay in treatment inevitably causes damage to the optic nerve head and subsequent permanent loss of vision. Because surgical treatment will be required the patient should be admitted to hospital and general measures taken to relieve the pain such as intravenous or intramuscular analgesics and anti-emetics for any nausea. The first aid treatment consists of instilling miotics in the form of Pilocarpine 2–4% eye drops intensively into the affected eye every 5 minutes for half an hour and then every 15 minutes for a further 2–3 hours. Intravenous Diamox (acetazolamide) 500 mg is given initially and if required also an intravenous infusion of mannitol to produce an osmotic diuresis. After a few hours the attack may be aborted and the definitive surgical treatment of peripheral iridectomy carried out at a convenient time. Should the acute attack of glaucoma not respond to this first aid treatment in a few hours surgical peripheral iridectomy should be carried out at once.

It should be stressed that the second eye frequently undergoes an attack of acute glaucoma within a few weeks and so a prophylactic peripheral iridectomy operation or laser iridotomy is performed on the unaffected eye at the time of the patient's admission to hospital.

Although surgical iridectomy is still the most widely used treatment Yag laser iridotomy is increasingly being used.

Congenital glaucoma (buphthalmos)

The name buphthalmos is applied to congenital glaucomas because of the huge enlargement of the eyes giving an impression of the eyes of cattle (ox eye—buphthalmos). It is uncommon but requires early recognition because of the serious visual outlook in an infant.

Most cases of buphthalmos are bilateral (66%) and most cases occur in boys (66%). The signs are:
1. Enlarged eyes
2. Watering of the eye with photophobia
3. Clouding of the corneas

Photophobia may cause the baby or infant to turn away from light and bury his head in the pillow. These signs may be noticed immediately at birth or any time during the first few months of life. Clouding of the corneas is due to corneal oedema and enlarged eyes are due to the raised intraocular pressure causing stretching of the cornea and sclera.

Treatment

Surgical operation undertaken at once is the only form of effective treatment. The principle of the operations is to fashion a gap in the abnormal mesoderm tissue in the angle of the anterior chamber (goniotomy) or to fashion a new outflow channel for aqueous (trabeculectomy) (Fig. 12.12).

SECONDARY GLAUCOMAS

A rise of intraocular pressure in one or both eyes is a common complication of other eye disease and sometimes systemic disease, therefore treatment is directed at the underlying condition. Some important causes of secondary glaucomas are as follows:

Fig. 12.12
Binocular congenital glaucoma

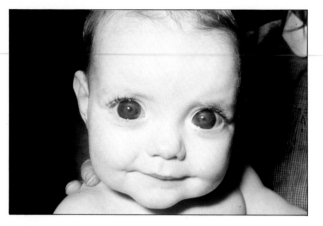

Iritis

Inflammatory cells from the inflamed iris obstruct the outflow of aqueous through the trabecular meshwork thus elevating the intraocular pressure. Prompt and effective treatment of the iritis usually alleviates this complication.

Injury

Injury, especially following intraocular haemorrhage and subluxation of the crystalline lens, may cause a rise of intraocular pressure by several mechanisms, such as obstruction to the aqueous outflow by blood cells, vitreous or direct damage to the angle of the anterior chamber.

Central retinal vein thrombosis

This particular type of secondary glaucoma supervenes in some patients some 3 months or so after a central retinal vein occlusion and is called neovascular (also called haemorrhagic or thrombotic) glaucoma. New blood vessels are formed in the angle of the anterior chamber giving rise to complete loss of vision which for practical purposes is untreatable. The condition is very painful requiring analgesics and sometimes leading to such severe distress for the patient that the blind and painful eye requires removal (Fig. 12.13).

Fig. 12.13
Neovascular glaucoma

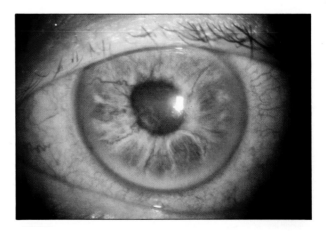

Steroid eye drops

In some individuals, long term treatment with steroid eye drops, for example in iritis, may lead to a secondary rise in intraocular pressure and the development of glaucoma. These individuals are called 'steroid eye responders' and the drops should be avoided in their case except under specialist supervision.

Pseudo-exfoliation of the lens capsule

A curious 'fluffing' of the lens capsule called pseudo-exfoliation, may cause secondary glaucoma (glaucoma capsulare). The areas affected give rise to two white ring opacities on the lens capsule. The condition is widespread in the population after middle-age, discovered mainly on routine examinations, and has an especially high incidence in Scandinavia. Treatment of an associated secondary glaucoma is exactly similar to that in chronic simple glaucoma (Fig. 12.14).

Fig. 12.14
Pseudo-exfoliation of lens capsule

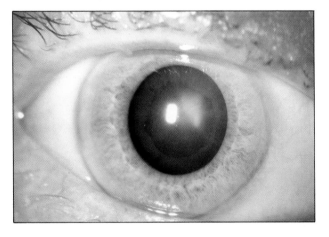

13

Orbital disease

ANATOMY

Disease of the orbital tissues will cause forward protrusion of the eyeball as the bony orbital walls are rigid (Fig. 13.1).

Protrusion of the eyeball is termed *proptosis* or *exophthalmos* and these terms have come to be synonymous. More precisely exophthalmos is protrusion of the eyeball alone and so is reserved for the protrusion found in dysthyroid disease, whereas proptosis is protrusion of the eyeball plus orbital contents as found in orbital tumours etc.

Fig. 13.1
Bones of the orbit

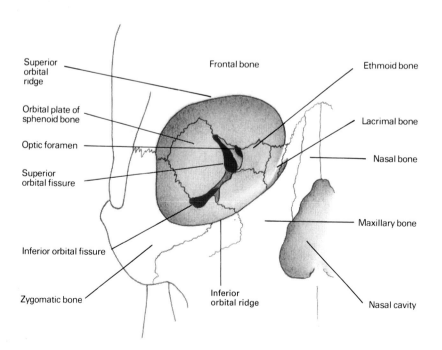

PARTICULAR FEATURES IN THE EXAMINATION OF ORBITAL DISEASE

The *degree of protrusion* is measured by observing the patient from behind and above, gently retracting the upper eyelids and comparing the anterior surfaces of the two corneas (Fig. 13.2).

An exophthalmometer may be used to give a precise measurement of the degree of protrusion.

Displacement of the eyeball upwards or downwards as well as the protrusion can best be observed by holding a horizontal rule across the face comparing the corneal margins on each side (Fig. 13.3).

Fig. 13.2
Examining for exophthalmos

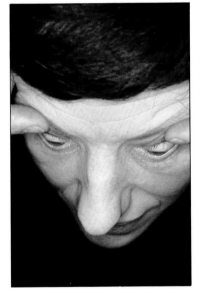

Fig. 13.3
Examination for displacement of the eye

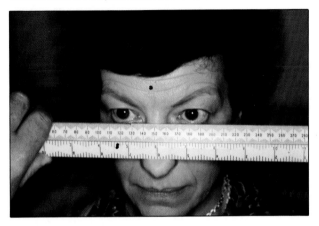

The orbital disease will be described under the following headings:
1. Dysthyroid disease
2. Orbital inflammation (or cellulitis)
3. Carotid-cavernous fistula
4. Orbital neoplasms

DYSTHYROID DISEASE

This refers to patients with excess or reduced thyroid hormone secretion. Characteristic appearances in the orbital regions occur both with hyperthyroidism and hypothyroidism.

Hyperthyroidism (thyrotoxicosis or Graves's disease)
The 'staring' appearance of patients with hyperthyroidism is due to exophthalmos and upper eyelid retraction, which in turn results from infiltration of the orbital tissues with lymphocytes and associated oedema. As well as the general signs of hyperthyroidism, i.e. increased pulse rate, excess sweating, weight loss and hand tremor, there are characteristic orbital *signs* as follows:

1. Exophthalmos: This is usually symmetrical between the two eyes but may be markedly asymmetrical giving rise to the impression of uni-ocular exophthalmos

2. Upper eyelid retraction: A characteristic sign of the hyperthyroidism, probably due to contraction of the smooth muscle component of the levator palpebrae superioris muscle (sympathetic nerve innervation). This retraction reveals a white rim of sclera at the upper corneal margin.

3. Lid lag: When the eyes look downwards there is a delay in the normal associated downward movement of the upper eyelid

4. Defective eye movement: Single or multiple ocular muscles may show defective movement giving rise to diplopia in certain positions of gaze. The superior rectus muscles seem to be most often affected (Fig. 13.4).

Fig. 13.4
Thyrotoxicosis with exophthalmos, eyelid retraction and defective eye movement

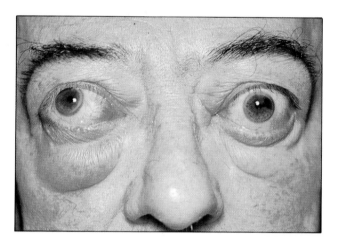

Discomfort of the eyes from corneal and conjunctival exposure often occurs with exophthalmos and upper eyelid retraction. Lubricant eye drops as required may be used (e.g. Hypromellose eye drops) and the eyelid retraction may be lessened using guanethidine sulphate 5% (Ismelin) eye drops once or twice a day.

Severe and progressive exophthalmos occasionally occurs ('malignant exophthalmos') in hyperthyroidism causing extreme protrusion of the eyes, gross periorbital oedema and inability to close the eyelids. In such cases urgent measures to protect the cornea are essential. These include tarsorrhaphy (suturing together of the eyelids partially or completely) and surgical decompression of the orbits.

Hypothyroidism (myxoedema)

Ocular signs of hypothyroidism, less common except in the late stages of the disease, are swelling of the eyelids without any reddening of the skin and occasionally exophthalmos (Fig. 13.5).

Fig. 13.5
Myxoedema

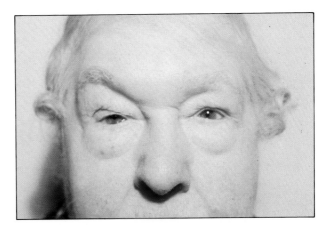

ORBITAL INFLAMMATION (OR CELLULITIS)

Inflammation of the orbital tissues is usually caused by *spread of infection*, mostly bacterial, *from adjacent structures* in and around the orbit. Thus orbital cellulitis may occur as a direct spread of infection from any of the paranasal air sinuses (especially the thin-walled ethmoid sinuses) and the lacrimal gland. Injuries to the orbit may also introduce infection.

Signs
1. Severe redness of the skin
2. Swelling of the eyelids
3. Protrusion of the eye
4. Purulent discharge from the hyperaemic conjunctiva
5. Pain which may be severe (Fig. 13.6)

The danger of orbital cellulitis lies in its potential damage to the optic nerve and the spread of infection to cause meningitis. Orbital and paranasal air sinus X-rays should be taken as soon as practicable.

Treatment
Systemic broad-spectrum antibiotics should be given at once. Bacterial cultures of any purulent ocular or periorbital discharge may indicate a specific organism with staphylococcus being the most common. Analgesics for the pain should be given as required. Failure of the orbital cellulitis to respond within 48 hours or less of treatment is an indication for the patient to be admitted to hospital for intravenous antibiotic infusion.

Once the orbital cellulitis has settled sufficiently any underlying sinus infection may require definitive surgical treatment.

Fig. 13.6
Orbital cellulitis

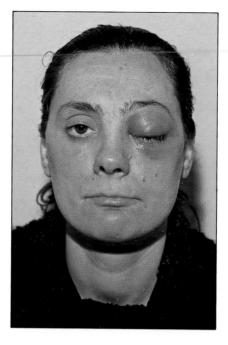

CAROTID-CAVERNOUS FISTULA

Carotid artery aneurysms may rupture spontaneously, or as a result of trauma, into the cavernous sinus. The carotid arterial blood thus refluxes into the venous blood of the cavernous sinus giving rise to a carotid-cavernous fistula.

Symptoms
1. Rapid onset of throbbing orbital pain
2. Protrusion of the eye
3. Blurred vision
A head injury may have preceded the symptoms.

Signs
1. Pulsating exophthalmos
2. Protrusion of the eye
3. Swelling of the eyelids
4. Marked dilatation of the vessels in the eye
5. Vision is impaired
6. Auscultation reveals a loud bruit over the orbit
Investigations to confirm the diagnosis are carotid arteriography and computerised tomography (CT) scan (Fig. 13.7).

Treatment
Spontaneous resolution of the carotid-cavernous fistula occurs in a proportion of cases over several years. Where vision is threatened or the exophthalmos is progressive or intolerable then surgical ligation of the common or internal carotid artery may be required.

Fig. 13.7
Carotid-cavernous fistula: note eye
protrusion and dilatation of vessels.
(Courtesy of the Western Ophthalmic
Hospital)

Fig. 13.8
Orbital tumour

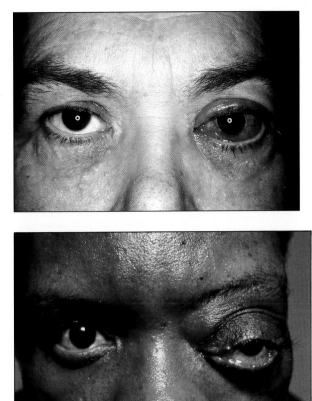

ORBITAL NEOPLASMS (FIG. 13.8)

Several primary and secondary neoplasms may arise within the orbit
or adjacent structures and are as follows:

Primary neoplasms
1. Haemangioma
2. Lymphomas (including reticuloses, leukaemia and Hodgkin's
   disease deposits)
3. Glioma of the optic nerve
4. Neurofibroma
5. Meningioma (usually arising from the sphenoidal ridge)
6. Dermoid cyst
7. Lacrimal gland adenoma and adenoid cystic carcinoma
8. Osteogenic sarcoma

Secondary neoplasms
1. Metastatic tumours arising from primary carcinoma of the breast
   and lung in particular
2. Nasopharyngeal and sinus carcinomas extending into the orbit
3. Intraocular tumours spreading into the orbit (malignant melanoma of choroid and retinoblastoma).

Symptoms
1. Protrusion of the eye
2. Blurring of vision
3. Aching pain in the orbit
4. Diplopia

Signs
1. Proptosis (and displacement of the eye in one direction depending on the site of the tumour)
2. Reduced vision from optic nerve compression
3. Defective eye movements giving squint and diplopia
4. Periorbital oedema and hyperaemia with rapidly growing tumours

Particular clinical features and investigations aiding diagnosis of orbital neoplasms

Age
Epidermoid cysts of the orbit, retinoblastoma extending into the orbit; osteogenic sarcoma; optic nerve glioma and orbital neuro-fibroma occur predominantly in infants and children.

Metastatic orbital tumours are more common after middle-age, and meningioma in the 25–40 years age group.

Direction of eye displacement
A tumour will displace the eyeball laterally or vertically when it arises at the side of the eyeball. For example a neurofibroma in the upper orbital tissue will cause downward displacement and a lacrimal gland adenocarcinoma will displace the eyeball inwards (medially).

Systemic features
A careful history and systemic examination will indicate the possibility of a primary tumour elsewhere. Associated systemic features should be sought, e.g. the 'cafe au lait' skin spots on the trunk of multiple neurofibromatosis (von Recklinghausen's disease) suggesting an orbital neurofibroma; and general enlargement of lymph nodes indicating Hodgkin's disease or leukaemia.

Investigations
1. Full blood count: Anaemia and abnormal white cell counts will be a feature of leukaemia and Hodgkin's disease in particular
2. Chest X-ray: Primary lung carcinomas, enlarged hilar lymph nodes and reticuloses will be revealed
3. Orbital and skull X-rays: Direct visualisation of a meningioma (of the sphenoidal ridge in particular) and enlargement of the optic foramen (optic nerve glioma) may sometimes be possible with plain X-rays.
4. Ultrasonography: An orbital tumour may be outlined by ultrasound scan.
5. Computerised tomography (CT) scan: Delineation of the site and size of an orbital tumour is usually possible with the CT scan (Fig. 13.9).

Fig. 13.9
CT scan of head: note proptosis of left eye and tumour in lateral and posterior orbit. (Lacrimal gland adenoid cystic carcinoma)

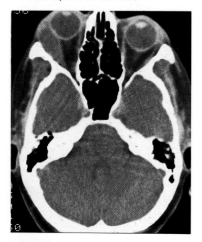

6. Magnetic resonance imaging (MRI): Clearer resolution of an orbital or adjacent tumour is possible with MRI and this must now be regarded as essential for accurate diagnosis (Fig. 13.10).

Treatment

Localised progressive orbital tumours usually require surgical removal retaining the eye whenever possible. For rapidly growing malignant primary and secondary malignant tumours chemotherapy and radiotherapy will be required.

Fig. 13.10
Parasagittal MRI of head showing mucocele in roof of orbit. (Courtesy of Dr G. Lloyd)

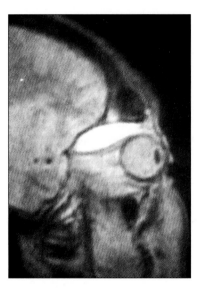

14

Fundus conditions

ANATOMY

The *normal fundus oculi,* when observed with the ophthalmoscope, varies a little between individuals in the background colour (due to variations in retinal pigment) but the optic disc and vessels are remarkably uniform.

The *background reddish-orange colour* of the fundus is due to the retinal pigment epithelial layer overlying the choroid. Sparse pigmentation will allow choroidal vessels to be seen in the fundus. Heavy pigmentation, seen in Asian and African races, gives a deep reddish-orange colour and also a tigroid appearance (likened to a tiger's stripes!). The retina itself is transparent hence the background reddish-orange colour of the pigment epithelial layer and choroid is observed *through* the retina.

The *optic disc* is the prominent feature of the fundus situated just nasal to the central area of the fundus (the macula). It is slightly oval in shape and marks the commencement of the optic nerve. Fine capillaries cover its surface giving it a lighter red colour contrasted with the darker fundus colour. The disc has clear margins and in its centre a depression called the *physiological cup* (Fig. 14.1, 14.2)

Fig. 14.1
The fundus

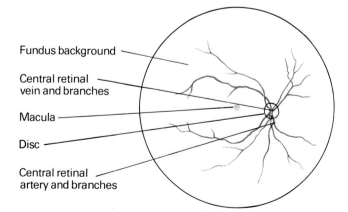

Fundus background

Central retinal vein and branches

Macula

Disc

Central retinal artery and branches

Fig. 14.2
Histological section through the retina

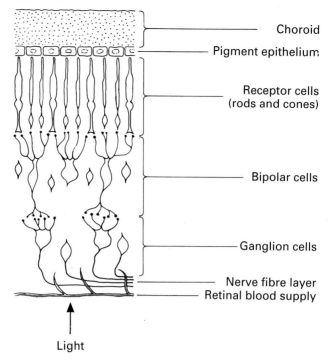

Choroid

Pigment epithelium

Receptor cells
(rods and cones)

Bipolar cells

Ganglion cells

Nerve fibre layer
Retinal blood supply

Light

The *retinal blood vessels* are observable directly with the ophthalmoscope, the only site in the body where this can be achieved. The veins (or more accurately venules) are observed as columns of bluish blood in transparent vessel walls carrying de-oxygenated blood *to* the central retinal vein at the disc. The arteries (more accurately arterioles) are narrower than the veins and appear as red columns of blood in transparent walls carrying oxygenated blood *away* from the optic disc to supply the retina.

The *macula* is the centre feature of the fundus. It appears as a darker red spot on the surrounding fundus with a bright centre point which is the reflected ophthalmoscope light from the minute pit marking the fovea (Fig. 14.3, 14.4, 14.5).

Fig. 14.3
The normal fundus

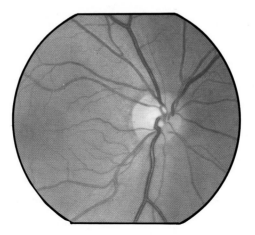

Fig. 14.4
The normal fundus: painting

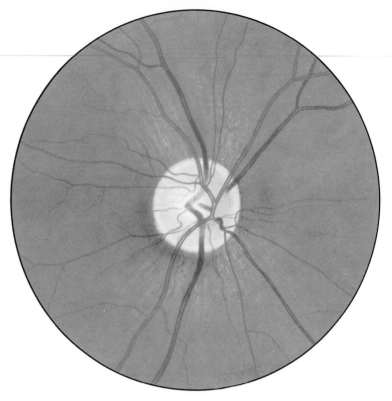

Fig. 14.5
The macular region of the normal
fundus

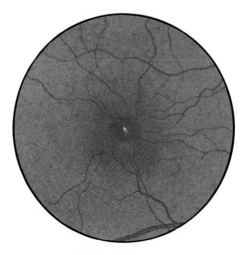

The following fundus conditions will be described:
1. Congenital fundus anomalies
   Opaque retinal nerve fibres
   Myopic crescent
2. Vascular fundus conditions
   Arteriosclerosis
   Hypertension
   Central retinal artery occlusion
   Central retinal vein occlusion
   Blood dyscrasias
   Diabetes mellitus and diabetic retinopathy
3. Senile macular degeneration
4. Retinal detachment
5. Fundus inflammation
   Choroiditis and chorioretinitis
6. Fundus neoplasms
   Benign melanoma of the choroid
   Malignant melanoma of the choroid
   Retinoblastoma
   Secondary tumours
7. Retinal dystrophies
   Retinitis pigmentosa
   Macular dystrophy

CONGENITAL FUNDUS ANOMALIES

Opaque retinal nerve fibres
Retinal nerve fibres are normally non-myelinated but occasionally the myelin sheaths of the optic nerve fibres extend on to the retina as a congenital anomaly.

This is seen as a bright white patch adjacent to the disc often obscuring the retinal vessels running in the white patch. Its importance lies in recognising the appearance as a harmless anomaly and is invariably noted on routine examination of the fundus (Fig. 14.6).

Myopic crescent
In congenital and acquired myopia a crescent of white with black pigmented borders may be observed next to the disc. The crescent is usually temporal to the disc but may completely surround it. In pathological myopia the myopic crescent will be associated with myopic choroidoretinal degeneration. This crescent is a rim of atrophic choroid revealing the underlying white sclera in a crescent shape (Fig. 14.7).

Fig. 14.6
Opaque or myelinated retinal nerve
fibres

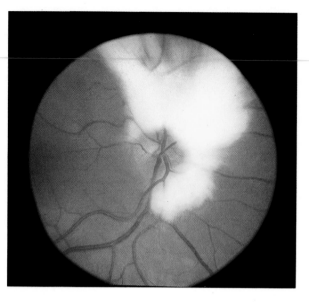

Fig. 14.7
Myopic crescent: note prominent
choroidal vessels often seen in
myopia (Courtesy of the Western
Ophthalmic Hospital)

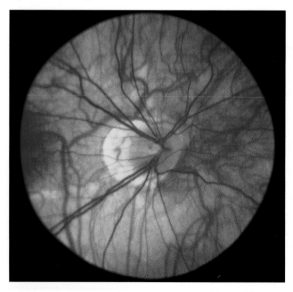

Fig. 14.8
Normal fluorescein angiography (late
venous phase) showing normal
pattern of vessels

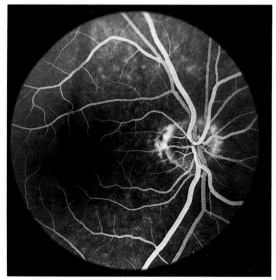

VASCULAR FUNDUS CONDITIONS

Fluorescein angiography of the retina

This technique allows a detailed recorded examination of retinal vascular structure. It is performed by injecting 5 ml of 10% fluorescein solution into the antecubital vein of the patient and then taking a series of monochrome photographs of the fundus in rapid succession about every second. This records the flow of fluorescein through the retinal circulation as it passes in succession through arterioles, capillaries and venules. It demonstrates more clearly than normal ophthalmoscopy details such as vascular occlusions, leaking abnormal capillaries, microaneurysms and retinal oedema.

Fluorescein angiography is especially valuable in diabetic retinopathy and other retinal vascular disease and choroidal neoplasms (Fig. 14.8, 14.9).

Arteriosclerosis

The changes associated with arteriosclerosis of retinal blood vessels must be regarded as normal and universally seen in the fundi of old people. It is important to recognise these appearances in order to distinguish them from the fundus changes of hypertension. They carry *no visual symptoms* for the patient. Slight narrowing of the retinal arteries giving a brighter reflection of light from the artery surface (the vessel light 'reflex' or reflection), and an irregular calibre of the arterial walls are the principal fundus signs. Nipping of the arterio-venous crossing may also be seen near the disc (Fig. 14.10).

Fig. 14.9
Diabetic fluorescein angiography demonstrating microaneurysms as brightly fluorescing spots

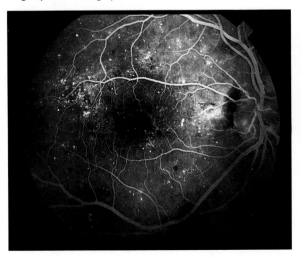

Fig. 14.10
Arteriosclerosis of the retinal vessels

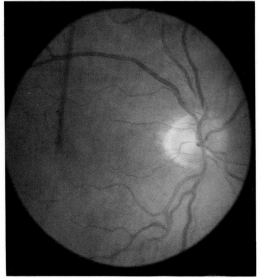

Hypertension

Systemic vascular hypertension, from whatever cause, will produce important diagnostic fundus appearances which are carefully monitored during the general examination and follow-up of patients with this condition. These appearances vary with the severity and duration of the hypertension and are best described under the three headings of mild, moderate and severe.

Mild or early hypertensive fundus appearance

This is largely a more obvious version of the normal subtle arteriosclerotic fundus change. The arteries are narrowed and tortuous giving a bright reflection of light from the artery surface. (The terms 'copper-wire' arteries and 'silver-wire' arteries are rather confusing since copper to one observer may be silver to another! These terms indicate the relative brightness of the ophthalmoscope light reflected in relation to the width of the artery wall. It is better to refer to retinal artery narrowing as mild, moderate and marked.)

Arterio-venous nipping may be seen wherever an artery crosses over a vein and is due to the thickened arterial wall compressing the underlying vein thus tapering off the column of blood in that part of the vein (Fig. 14.11).

Fig. 14.11
Early hypertension: note arterio-venous (a-v) nipping and arteriolar narrowing

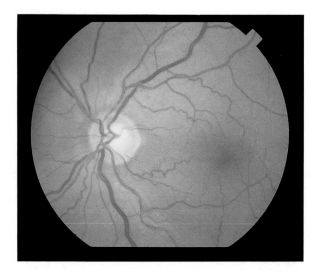

Moderate hypertensive fundus appearance

As well as arterial narrowing, tortuosity and arterio-venous nipping two additional signs may be seen in the fundi of moderate hypertensives. These are haemorrhages and soft exudates. The *haemorrhages are flame shaped* because they conform to the retinal nerve fibres running across the superficial retina. They slowly absorb if hypertensive treatment is adequate. The *soft exudates* or '*cotton-wool*' *spots* represent acute arterial occlusions (infarcts) of the retina and appear rapidly. The cotton-wool spot appearance is due to interruption of axoplasmic flow in the retinal nerve fibres; the subsequent build up of transported material giving the white appearance. Over many weeks the fluffy cotton-wool spot will absorb by phagocytosis. The appearance of these spots gives rise to concern in hypertension as it often indicates inadequate control of the hypertension and possible similar vascular damage of other tissues especially the kidneys and brain (Fig. 14.12).

Fig. 14.12
Moderate hypertension: note haemorrhages and cotton-wool spots

Fig. 14.13
Severe hypertension: note the swollen disc in addition to vessel changes and haemorrhages

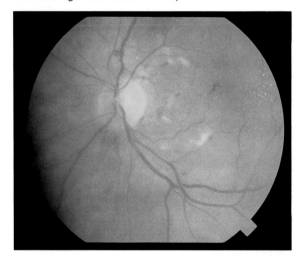

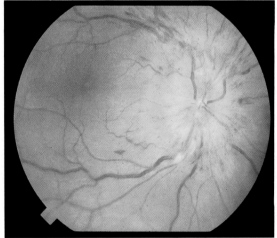

Severe (malignant or accelerated) hypertension
Rapid onset hypertension especially in young people may be accompanied by blurring of vision as a presenting symptom.

The fundus signs in severe hypertension consist of the milder hypertensive signs in greater degree plus the additional sign of *papilloedema*. When papilloedema occurs the term *malignant hypertension* is used to indicate the gravity of the situation and the threat to the patient's life from a cerebro-vascular accident in particular.

Thus, marked arterial narrowing, marked arterio-venous nipping, large numbers of flame shaped haemorrhages, large numbers of soft exudates (cotton-wool spots) and papilloedema constitute the fundus signs of severe hypertension. With these signs the patient should be admitted at once to hospital for control of the hypertension (Fig. 14.13).

Central retinal artery occlusion

Sudden loss of vision in the affected eye ocurs with central artery occlusion and is profound, with perception of light only remaining. It is in effect infarction of the inner two-thirds of the retina (nerve fibre layer, ganglion and bipolar cells). Recovery is very rare as the central retinal artery is an end artery to the retina which itself is part of the central nervous system. Once the blood supply to the retina has been obstructed for more than an hour or two permanent destruction of the retinal cells occurs with consequent loss of function. An embolus (from carotid artery or heart) or a thrombus is the usual cause of retinal artery occlusion.

Causes are particularly hypertension, atrial fibrillation, carotid artery stenosis, blood dyscrasias and diabetes mellitus. Investigations should be directed on these lines.

The *signs* are perception of light only, a reduced or absent direct pupil light reflex and the characteristic fundus appearance. A few hours after the event the central fundus looks slightly paler than normal (due to ischaemic retinal swelling hence obscuring the normal reddish-orange background choroid colour) and (for the same reason) the macula looks relatively bright red in contrast (the *'cherry red' spot*). The retinal arteries are very narrowed. These fundus signs subside over 6–8 weeks to be replaced by a normal fundus background but a very pale disc (*optic atrophy*).

A *branch retinal artery occlusion* will produce the same fundus signs but they are confined to the quadrant of supply of the particular branch artery. (Fig. 14.14, 14.15).

Fig. 14.14
Central retinal artery occlusion: note cherry red spot (Courtesy of Western Ophthalmic Hospital)

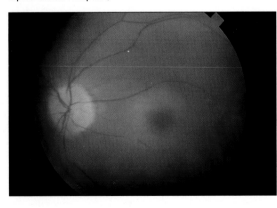

Fig. 14.15
Inferior branch retinal artery occlusion

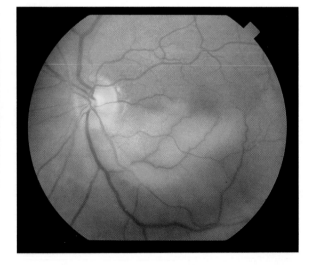

Aetiology of central and branch retinal artery occlusion is: embolisation (especially particles of atheroma from the major arteries particularly the carotid arteries. One indication for carotid artery vascular surgery is central retinal artery occlusion from the emboli of atheroma)

cranial arteritis (temporal or giant-cell arteritis) (see page 129)

sickle cell disease and other blood dyscrasias

retrobulbar haemorrhage

dysthyroid exophthalmos

Treatment

Retinal artery occlusion is a medical emergency. Urgent treatment is worthwhile if the patient presents within a few hours of the event. Methods to improve retinal blood flow and to dislodge an embolus are gentle digital massage of the eye through the upper eyelid, inhalation of 95% oxygen–5% carbon dioxide mixture, intravenous acetazolamide and paracentesis. Paracentesis is the surgical release of aqueous with a fine needle to rapidly lower ocular pressure.

Transient blurring of vision (amaurosis fugax) which may last seconds or hours is a serious symptom and requires investigation as to an underlying cause listed above.

Central retinal vein occlusion

Sudden loss of vision in the affected eye occurs with an occlusion of the central retinal vein and is usually to a level of 6/60 or less. In a few cases some recovery of vision may occur over several months (in contrast to central retinal artery occlusion). A thrombus is the usual cause of the occlusion.

Causes are hypertension, diabetes mellitus and blood dyscrasias. Investigations should be directed to these causes in particular also investigating for primary malignant disease which can be associated with generalised thrombotic episodes.

The *signs* are reduced vision to approximately 6/60 or less, reduced direct pupil light reflex and characteristic fundus signs. The fundus signs are marked *dilatation and tortuosity of the retinal veins, haemorrhages* over the whole fundus extending to the periphery, *scattered soft exudates* and *swelling of the optic disc*. These signs are all due to rupture of small capillaries with the reduced venous blood flow and ischaemic disc oedema (Fig. 14.16, 14.17).

Over several months the signs will gradually disappear and some improvement in vision may occur. Permanent residual fundus signs of abnormal tortuous vessel loops may remain in the fundus.

Neovascular (thrombotic or haemorrhagic) glaucoma may occur three months approximately after a central retinal vein occlusion (see Ch. 12) as a severe and intractable complication.

A *branch retinal vein occlusion* will produce the same fundus signs but confined to the quadrant of the fundus corresponding to the occluded vein.

Fig. 14.16
Central retinal vein occlusion
(Courtesy of Western Ophthalmic
Hospital)

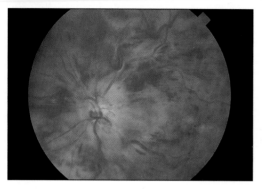

Fig. 14.17
Superior branch retinal vein occlusion

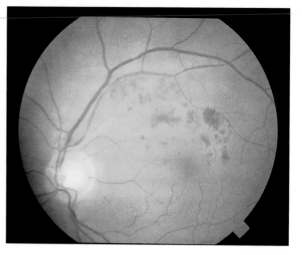

Treatment of central retinal or branch vein occlusion should be directed at any underlying *cause*, e.g. hypertension.

Pan-retinal laser photo-coagulation is effective in markedly reducing the complication of neovascular glaucoma.

Blood dyscrasias

Anaemia and leukaemia
Any profound anaemia and leukaemia may cause visual failure from either retinal haemorrhages or from central retinal vein and artery occlusions. The fundus signs are of haemorrhages and soft exudates (cotton-wool spots) *without* retinal vessel signs (Fig. 14.18).

Sickle-cell disease
Amongst African and descendent races abnormal haemoglobins may be found as an inherited disorder. They may be distinguished by blood haemoglobin electrophoresis and are designated haemoglobin S and C (called sickle cell trait) when in a heterozygous individual but SS, CC and SC in homozygous individuals (sickle cell disease or anaemia).

Visual failure occurs from retinal haemorrhages particularly in sickle cell SC disease but can also occur in the other varieties of abnormal haemoglobin. Peripheral retinal vascular occlusions cause retinal and vitreous haemorrhages, new retinal vessel tufts and white glial or fibrous strands which can lead to traction retinal detachment (Fig. 14.19).

Treatment
Laser photocoagulation of the retina in sickle cell disease may be required to coagulate new vessels.

Fig. 14.18
Fundus in leukaemia

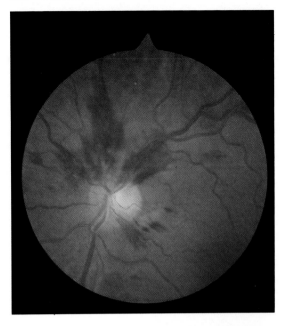

Fig. 14.19
Fundus in sickle cell disease

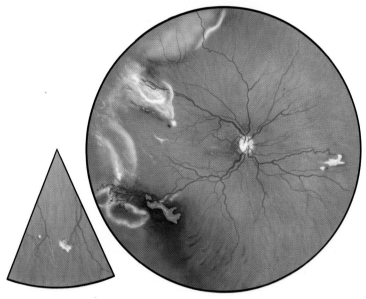

Diabetes mellitus and diabetic retinopathy

Diabetic patients are prone to *eyelid styes*, the formation of eyelid *xanthelasma*, earlier development of *senile cataracts* and specific retinal damage called *diabetic retinopathy*.

The development of diabetic retinopathy is related to two factors:

1. The duration of diabetes; diabetic retinopathy may be observed in approximately 80% of diabetics after 20 years of the disease

2. The control of the diabetes; adequate control delays or lessens the development of diabetic retinopathy

Diabetic retinopathy may usefully be classified into the following two types:

1. Background: the lesions are located mainly between the main temporal vessels and are within the retina layers
2. Proliferative: new vessels appear on the surface of the retina or within the vitreous
3. Mixed: a combination of these two

Symptoms

Gradual or rapid visual deterioration may occur. Vitreous haemorrhage or macular haemorrhage will cause sudden loss of vision.

Signs

The severity of the signs in the retina increase with the duration of the diabetes. They are: dilation of veins, microaneurysms, 'blot' haemorrhages, hard exudates and new vessels.

The microaneurysms appear as fine red dots, frequently in clusters. 'Blot' haemorrhages occur as a result of the microaneurysms rupturing and appear as red blobs in the fundus. Hard exudates take several years to form and usually take 6 months to become visible. These hard exudates are yellow deposits of lipids and coalesce together to form larger ones over the years (background diabetic retinopathy). New vessels may form on the retina or extend into the vitreous causing further retinal and vitreous haemorrhages (proliferative diabetic retinopathy) (Fig. 14.20, 14.21).

Fig. 14.20
Moderate diabetic retinopathy: note hard exudates, haemorrhages and microaneurysms

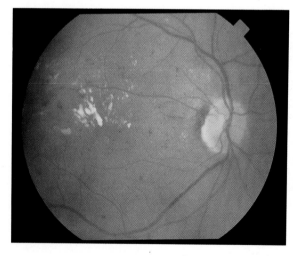

Fig. 14.21
Late diabetic retinopathy

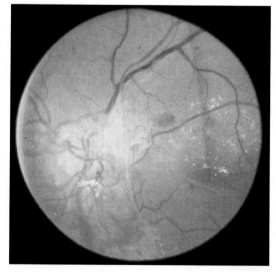

The visual acuity falls rapidly when the macula is involved (diabetic maculopathy) either with hard exudates, microaneurysms, haemorrhages and macular oedema.

Treatment

Diabetic retinopathy may be controlled by the following measures:

Adequate control of the diabetes.

Laser photocoagulation. The object of laser treatment, which can be carried out as an out-patient, is to destroy areas of new vessels and microaneurysms in the retina. Repeated treatments may be required over the years but recent work suggests early and adequate treatment improves the visual prognosis in diabetes considerably.

AGE-RELATED MACULAR DEGENERATION

Gradual deterioration of vision over several years and distortion of vision are the symptoms of this condition. As the name implies it is largely confined to the elderly and is one of the most common causes of registrable blindness in Western countries.

The fundus signs are usually symmetrical between the two eyes and consist of a granular pigmented and speckled area confined to the macular region.

No specific treatment is available (Fig. 14.22).

Colloid bodies (or *drusen*) are yellow spots scattered round the macular region and are often associated with pigment speckling at the macula. These colloid bodies are hyaline thickenings in Bruch's membrane of the choroid and may be seen in many patients long before there is visual deterioration due to the later associated macular pigmentary speckling (Fig. 14.23).

Fig. 14.22
Age-related macular degeneration

Fig. 14.23
Colloid bodies of the fundus

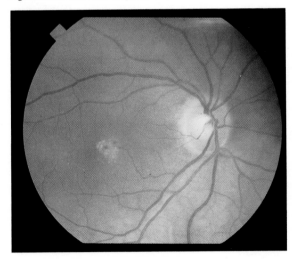

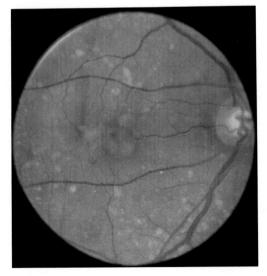

One variety is called *disciform macular degeneration* and may be very rapid in onset owing to choroid and macular haemorrhages occurring. If the diagnosis is made early enough then laser photo-coagulation treatment can sometimes be beneficial in arresting new capillaries developing in the subretinal layer.

RETINAL DETACHMENT

This is a condition in which the retina becomes separated from its pigment epithelial layer. The separation occurs at this site for embryological reasons: the two walls of the embryonic optic vesicle become apposed and form respectively the pigment epithelium of the retina and the neuro-retina. Retinal detachment is most common after the age of 50 years and is commonest in high myopia. Trauma plays a part in younger patients and in high myopes who have a predisposition.

A lower incidence is reported in African races.

Symptoms
Sudden onset of *floating specks* or spots associated with *flashes of light* in the affected eye are typical symptoms. The same day or days or weeks later a 'shadow' or 'curtain' in the visual field can be seen which gradually extends to cover the whole visual field.

Signs
Reduced visual acuity will be marked if the macular region becomes detached. There will be visual field loss corresponding to the area of detached retina, e.g. the temporal retina generally detaches first thereby giving a nasal field defect.

The detached retina may be seen with the ophthalmoscope as a greyish area and retinal folds which quiver as the eye moves. The blood vessels on the detached part of the retina appear as a deeper red colour than normal. If an area of retina still remains in situ an easy contrast between the normal fundus colour and the greyish detached portion can be observed.

A *retinal break* will be seen at the periphery of the detached fundus in the form of either a *tear* ('arrowhead' or 'U' shaped), a *hole* or a *dialysis*. The dialysis is particularly associated with trauma.

Careful examination of the fellow eye should be undertaken to search for symptomless retinal breaks (Fig. 14.24, 14.25).

Treatment
A retinal detachment operation is the only form of treatment possible. The principles of this operation are to seal the retinal break (tear, hole or dialysis) with cryotherapy and relieve the traction over the break by attaching to the sclera an indenting implant of silastic.

The visual prognosis depends on the duration of the detachment, the nature and number of retinal breaks and whether the macula has been detached.

Fig. 14.24
Arrowhead retinal tear and detachment

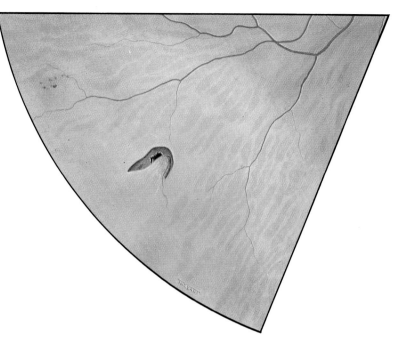

Fig. 14.25
Retinal detachment with retinal dialysis

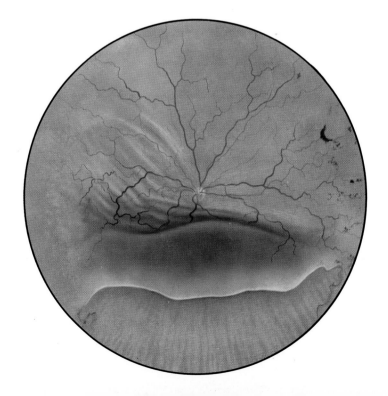

Prophylactic treatment of the fellow eye may be possible by cryotherapy or photocoagulation of a retinal tear not yet detached.

Asymptomatic retinal tears and holes may sometimes be seen on a routine examination of the fundus. Similarly, retinal tears may present with symptoms like those of a retinal detachment, namely floating opacities and flashing lights. Such tears will ultimately lead to a detachment of the retina within hours, weeks or months, but can be treated with laser photocoagulation or retinal cryotherapy *and thus prevent a retinal detachment* occurring. Hence the necessity to take urgent action with patients with these symptoms.

FUNDUS INFLAMMATION

Choroiditis (posterior uveitis) and chorioretinitis

Inflammation of the choroid causes rapid blurring of vision in usually one eye with 'spots' and 'haziness' over the whole visual field (due to inflammatory cells in the vitreous). Because the choroid and retina lie next to each other inflammation of the choroid always affects the overlying retina to produce a chorioretinitis.

The causes of choroiditis are listed below.

Toxoplasmosis

The toxoplasmosis parasite (a protozoan, *Toxoplasma gondii*) probably causes choroiditis by its entry into the bloodstream from ingested infected material from wild or domestic animals. The parasite may be transmitted across the placenta so that congenital toxoplasmosis may occur.

Many people are unaware they have had a toxoplasmosis chorioretinitis in childhood or from birth until a characteristic old fundus lesion is noted on routine examination in later years. Toxoplasmosis primary infection in adults may be accompanied by a mild febrile illness which precedes the eye symptoms.

The *signs* of active toxoplasmosis chorioretinitis are reduced vision, a very hazy view of the fundus (because of the inflammatory cells in the vitreous) and a localised white, fluffy area in the fundus often at the macula.

The fundus signs change as the chorioretinitis subsides over many weeks and finally there remains a heavily pigmented, circumscribed pale area of choroidal atrophy (Fig. 14.26, 14.27).

Treatment of toxoplasmosis chorioretinitis depends on visual impairment or its potential to cause visual loss. Treatment is usually commenced when there is a rapid decrease in vision which implies the inflammatory focus is at the macula or optic disc.

Combinations of oral treatment used are pyrimethamine (Daraprim, Maloprim), Sulphadiazine with or without clindamycin (Dalacin). Corticosteroids are also used with these drug combinations (e.g. Prednisolone tablets 40 mg per day in reducing dosage over several weeks) in order to reduce the inflammatory response in the retina to minimise scarring.

Fig. 14.26
Recurrence of choroiditis adjacent to old toxoplasmosis pigmented area of choroido-retinal atrophy

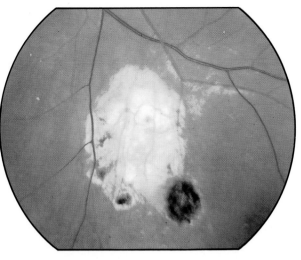

Fig. 14.27
Area of old, inactive choroiditis due to toxoplasmosis

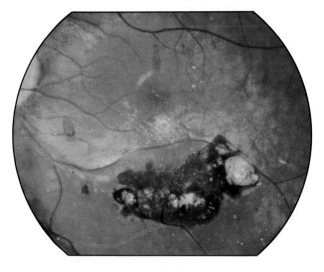

However, treatment is only required when the focus of chorio-retinitis threatens the macula or optic nerve (juxta-papillary choroiditis). Peripheral retinal foci of chorioretinitis may be left untreated as they do not threaten central vision and natural resolution may be awaited.

Toxocariasis
The dog tapeworm eggs, *Toxocara canis* may be ingested in children from infected excreta. The subsequent larvae may cause a focal choroiditis (Fig. 14.28).

Acquired immune deficiency syndrome (AIDS)
AIDS affects all body systems by profound disruption of the cell mediated immune system and is caused by the human immuno-deficiency virus (HIV). In immuno-compromised patients such as

Fig. 14.28
Toxocariasis choroiditis

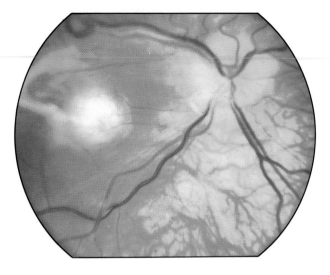

those with AIDS the cytomegalovirus (CMV) may produce an opportunistic *retinitis*. Patients with cytomegalovirus retinitis present with visual impairment and examination shows widespread areas of haemorrhage, occluded veins and white patches where there is active retinitis with infiltration of inflammatory cells in the retina (the 'tomato sauce and salad dressing' fundus, Fig. 14.29).

Fig. 14.29
Cytomegalovirus retinitis in AIDS ('tomato sauce and salad dressing' fundus) (Courtesy of Western Ophthalmic Hospital)

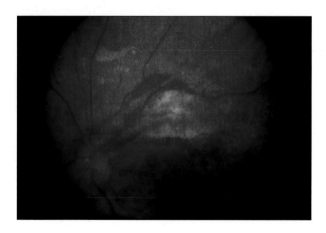

Other fundus manifestations of AIDS are 'cotton-wool' spots or soft exudates which represent acute arterial occlusions (infarcts) of the retinal arteries. They are not specific to AIDS and have the same aetiology as in other conditions, such as hypertension.

External eye infections in AIDS may also occur as opportunistic infections in the immuno-compromised individual, such as microsporidia kerato-conjunctivitis (an intracellular protozoan).

Histoplasmosis

This is a fungus infection endemic in some parts of North America. The choroiditis caused by this infection produces peripheral small areas of choroiditis but also may produce rapid visual loss because of macular haemorrhages.

Congenital syphilis

Usually only noticed on routine fundus examination and other signs of congenital syphilis will be present (saddle nose, alopecia, rhagades of the mouth, Hutchinson's teeth). The characteristic widespread old choroidoretinal patches of atrophy may be seen in the fundi.

FUNDUS NEOPLASMS

Benign melanoma of the choroid

Often called a choroidal naevus, a benign melanoma of the choroid is invariably *asymptomatic* and discovered only on routine ophthalmoscopic examination.

The ophthalmoscopic appearance is of a localised, flat, even, brown patch on the fundus. Benign melanomata are usually in the posterior pole of the fundus and about the size of the optic disc. There is no associated visual field defect (Fig. 14.30).

Fig. 14.30
Benign choroidal melanoma adjacent to disc

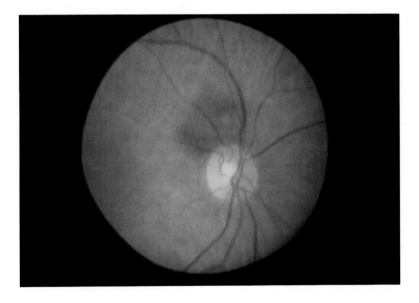

Once observed the melanoma should be kept under periodic review to establish that it is not enlarging, and also to establish that the rare change to a malignant melanoma has not occurred. Fundus photographs and fluorescein retinal angiography enable a clear record to be kept and aid diagnosis.

Malignant melanoma of the choroid

This primary malignant tumour of the choroid is most frequent in middle life.

Symptoms

Symptoms are similar to those of retinal detachment, namely an increasing 'shadow' or 'curtain' in the field of vision over a period of weeks. If a secondary retinal detachment occurs involving the macula, rapid visual loss will occur over a few days.

The ophthalmoscopic appearance is of a raised brown or grey area near the posterior pole of the fundus. With a large tumour there is frequently an associated secondary retinal detachment.

A visual field defect, corresponding to the site of the tumour, is present (Fig. 14.31).

Fig. 14.31
Malignant choroidal melanoma superiorly: note the raised vessels and greyish appearance

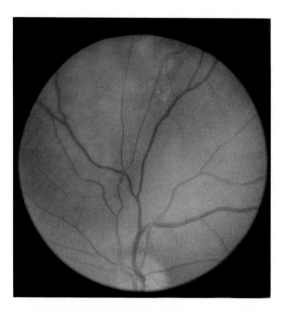

Fluorescein angiography of the fundus is an aid to diagnosis. Malignant melanoma metastasises widely in an unpredictable manner often after many years.

Magnetic resonance imaging (MRI) is also reliable in the diagnosis of malignant melanoma of the choroid (and other intraocular tumours) and may even demonstrate extraocular extension.

Treatment

Treatment is either removal of the affected eye or localised radiotherapy to the eye in the case of small tumours. There is some doubt whether early removal of the eye does affect the prognosis for life but clearly, where vision has been lost in an eye with a malignant melanoma, removal is desirable.

Fig. 14.32
Retinoblastoma

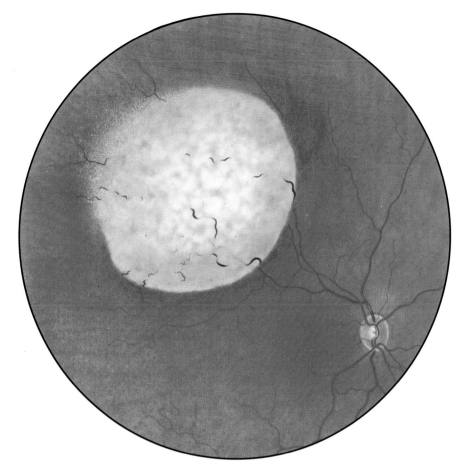

Retinoblastoma

This is the only primary malignant tumour of the retina and has its counterpart in the brain, the astrocytoma.

Retinoblastoma occurs in infants and most present within the first 2 years of life. The presenting symptoms noticed by the parents are a *white pupil* (the reflected light from the tumour has a white colour in the pupil) or a *squint*.

The ophthalmoscopic appearance is of a raised, white area in the fundus of the infant. There may be several tumours in one eye and bilateral tumours may also occur (Fig. 14.32).

Treatment

Treatment is removal of the eye if the retinoblastoma is large but localised radiotherapy to the eye may be used if the tumour is small.

A hereditary factor is present in retinoblastoma in many cases and an adult who has had a successfully treated retinoblastoma in childhood should receive sound genetic counselling in the event of him wishing to have children.

Secondary tumours

Primary tumours elsewhere in the body (especially carcinoma of the breast and bronchus) may give rise to secondary choroidal tumours. There is usually clinical evidence of the primary tumour site.

Blurred vision and a 'shadow' in the visual field will be noticed by the patient. The secondary choroidal tumour appears by ophthalmoscopy as a raised greyish-yellow area at the posterior pole of the fundus.

Treatment

Treatment of the secondary tumour in the choroid may occasionally be justified in the form of localised radiotherapy to the eye. However, the presence of a secondary choroidal tumour invariably indicates widespread metastases so that death occurs fairly soon after the diagnosis is made.

RETINAL DYSTROPHIES

Retinitis pigmentosa (primary pigmentary degeneration)

This condition is an *inherited* primary retinal degeneration. The mode of inheritance varies in different families and the severity of the disease also varies in families.

Symptoms

Night blindness in childhood or adolescence is the initial symptom. Following this there is gradual and progressive peripheral visual field loss leading eventually to 'tunnel vision'. The rate of progression varies greatly and in general the later the onset the less severe the final outcome.

Signs

Visual field loss in the early stages is characteristically in the form of a ring scotoma progressing later to total constriction of the visual fields ('tunnel vision') (Fig. 14.33, 14.34).

The fundus appearance shows the classical mid-periphery scattered pigmentation (likened to 'bone corpuscles'), marked narrowing of the retinal vessels and a pale disc (optic atrophy).

There is no known effective treatment but claims have been made from time to time of 'new' treatments. None have ever been substantiated unfortunately.

Macular dystrophy

Progressive degeneration of the maculae may occur in children and young adults occasionally as a hereditary disorder. There

Fig. 14.33
Retinitis pigmentosa

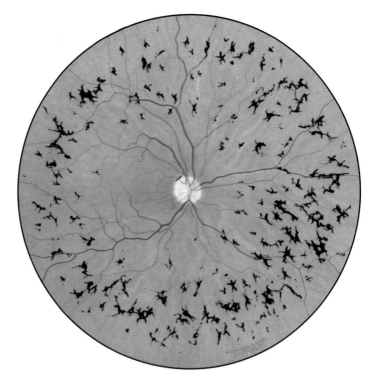

Fig. 14.34
Visual field defects of retinitis
pigmentosa

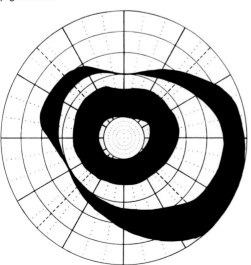

are several varieties of this disorder all leading to slow deterioration in central vision which may be noticed on routine vision screening in children or in young adults presenting with progressive visual failure.

The *signs* of this disorder are reduced visual acuities and a granular pigmentation at the maculae. No *treatment* is effective but special low vision aids (e.g. telescopic spectacles) may be of significant visual benefit and allow a normal education (Fig. 14.35).

Fig. 14.35
Macular dystrophy

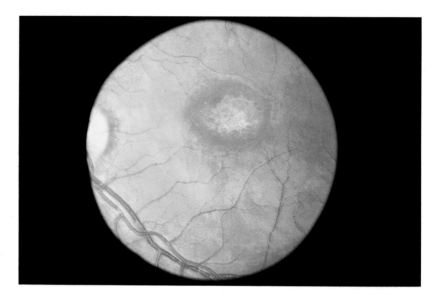

15

Optic nerve and visual pathway disorders

Damage to the optic nerve can be seen clinically with the ophthalmo-scope in the form of *papilloedema* (swelling of the optic disc) and *optic atrophy* (pallor of the optic disc).

Disorders of the optic chiasma, optic tract, optic radiations and visual (occipital) cortex manifest themselves with defects in the visual fields (Fig. 15.1).

Fig. 15.1
The visual pathway

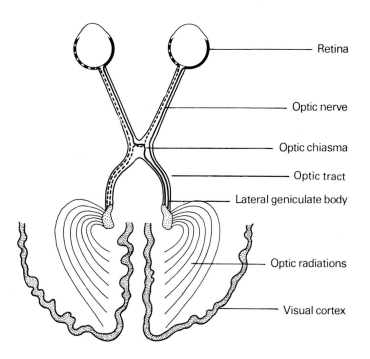

- Retina
- Optic nerve
- Optic chiasma
- Optic tract
- Lateral geniculate body
- Optic radiations
- Visual cortex

PAPILLOEDEMA

Swelling of the optic disc is produced by oedema within the nerve head. The causes of papilloedema are:

1. *Raised intracranial pressure:* Intracranial tumours cause raised intracranial pressure which in turn reduces venous outflow in the optic nerve head giving oedema of the optic disc.

2. *Ischaemia:* In hypertension, central retinal vein occlusion and cranial arteritis for example, reduced blood flow to the optic nerve head produces oedema.

3. *Inflammation:* This is called papillitis or optic neuritis and occurs in multiple sclerosis in particular.

The term papilloedema should really be restricted to a swollen optic disc due to raised intracranial pressure and it is probably better to refer to a swollen disc simply as such until the underlying cause is known.

Symptoms of the swollen disc
Whatever the cause, swelling of the optic disc causes blurring of vision to a variable extent which may be transient in raised intracranial pressure. Ischaemia of the disc in hypertension or cranial arteritis may cause very rapid and severe visual loss.

Signs of the swollen disc
1. Dilatation of the retinal veins
2. Blurred and raised disc margins
3. Reddish disc colour
4. The central physiological cup on the disc is filled in by oedema
5. Small haemorrhages at the disc margin
6. The pupil light reflex is reduced in conditions causing disc swelling
7. Enlarged blind spot on visual field plotting (Fig. 15.2)

Fig. 15.2
Swollen disc (papilloedema)

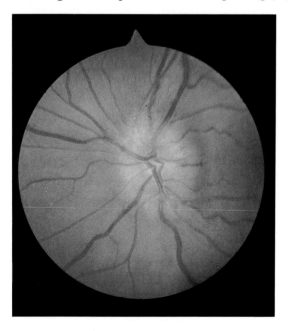

Conditions causing swollen discs

Intracranial tumours
Tumours in the posterior cranial fossa are particularly liable to cause papilloedema.

Hypertension
Disc swelling in hypertension will always be accompanied by the other fundus signs of hypertension. When disc swelling is present the term malignant hypertension is sometimes used (see Ch. 14).

Central retinal vein occlusion
Sudden loss of vision characterises an occlusion of the central retinal vein and the disc swelling will always be accompanied by the other fundus signs (see Ch. 14).

Cranial arteritis (temporal or giant-cell arteritis)
This condition is largely confined to the over 70s with sudden loss of vision in one or both eyes. The affected arteries may be any in the head and neck. Swelling of the optic disc with later optic atrophy and loss of vision occurs. The ESR (erythrocyte sedimentation rate) is raised. Other signs are tenderness on the scalp and prominent temporal arteries.

Systemic corticosteroid therapy should be initiated once the diagnosis has been confirmed in order to suppress the arteritis and prevent further vascular occlusions. After some months the corticosteroids may be gradually tailed off as the disease is self-limiting.

Multiple (disseminated) sclerosis (MS)
Most common in temperate climates this widespread neurological disease affects young adults mostly between the ages of 15–35 years and women are more commonly affected than men. Much evidence indicates that multiple sclerosis is a slow-virus infection of the nervous system. *Optic neuritis* is the main ophthalmological sign.

Rapid blurring of vision in one eye over a few hours is the presenting feature of many patients with MS. The vision falls to hand movements but peripheral vision is maintained. Gradual recovery of vision occurs over several weeks. *Pain on moving the eye* is present.

The *signs* of the optic neuritis of multiple sclerosis are:
1. Reduced visual acuity
2. Dense central scotoma
3. Diminished pupil light reflex
4. Swelling of the optic disc (papillitis or retrobulbar neuritis)
5. Two months after the onset a pale disc will supervene (optic atrophy)

Whilst the other signs are constant the disc swelling may not always be observed if the area of optic neuritis occurs well behind the optic disc. Hence *optic neuritis = retrobulbar neuritis* and if the optic nerve head is the part involved by the inflammation the alternative term *papillitis* may be used.

Other signs of multiple sclerosis may be present or follow later such as ataxia, parasthesiae and nystagmus.

OPTIC ATROPHY

Any damage to the optic nerve from whatever cause will result in degeneration of the optic nerve fibres and destruction of their myelin nerve sheaths. This may be observed clinically with the ophthalmoscope and is termed optic atrophy. Causal factors are:

1. *Ischaemia*: Following ischaemic disc swelling in hypertension and cranial arteritis, following central retinal artery occlusion and *especially* in chronic glaucoma
2. *Injury*: Direct injury of the orbit may cause severance or haemorrhage within the optic nerve
3. *Compression*: Tumours pressing on the optic nerve (see Ch. 13) and on the optic chiasma especially pituitary tumours
4. *Optic neuritis*: Associated with multiple sclerosis
5. *Toxins and nutrition*: Alcohol, tobacco, quinine toxicity and vitamin B deficiency
6. *Retinal degeneration*: Especially retinitis pigmentosa (see Ch. 14).

Signs of optic atrophy:
1. The disc is white overall or in part
2. The disc margins appear sharper because of the contrast between the pale disc and fundus colour
3. Diminished visual acuity
4. Visual field loss depending on the precise cause of the optic atrophy (Fig. 15.3)

Fig. 15.3
Optic atrophy

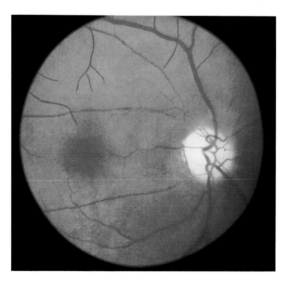

The history, visual field plotting, other associated signs and appropriate investigations will lead to an accurate assessment of the cause of the optic atrophy.

Toxic and nutritional optic atrophy

Very slow and progressive visual failure of both eyes with loss of colour vision occurs with poisoning by a number of toxic agents. The visual deterioration takes place over many months and even years.

Agents causing this slowly progressive optic atrophy are quinine and its derivatives (used as anti-malarials and for relieving night cramps), strong tobaccos and vitamin B deficiencies. It seems that certain individuals are prone to the toxic effects of tobacco especially when combined with high alcohol intake.

The signs of toxic and nutritional optic atrophy are diminished visual acuities, characteristic centro-caecal scotomata and pallor of the optic discs (Fig. 15.4).

Fig. 15.4
Centro-caecal scotoma field defect in toxic optic atrophy

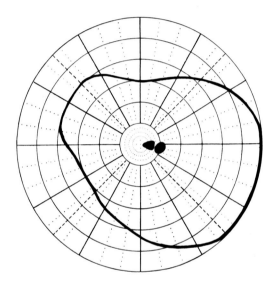

Treatment

Treatment consists of withdrawing the toxic agents, replacing any vitamin deficiency and a long term course of intramuscular injections of hydroxocobalamin (vitamin B_{12}) 1mg/three monthly after the four weekly initial loading doses.

PITUITARY TUMOURS: CHIASMAL COMPRESSION

Pituitary tumours are slowly expanding lesions (usually chromophobe adenomata) and because the optic chiasma lies immediately above the pituitary gland the chiasma is slowly compressed.

Visual symptoms of the chiasmal compression due to a pituitary tumour are of 'bumping into things' at the side and slight loss of visual acuity.

The *signs* are characteristic and consist of bilateral pale discs, reduced visual acuities and *bitemporal hemianopia* (commencing supero-temporally because of the initial compression of the underside of the optic chiasma) (Fig. 15.5).

Fig. 15.5
Bitemporal hemianopia visual field defect in chiasmal compression

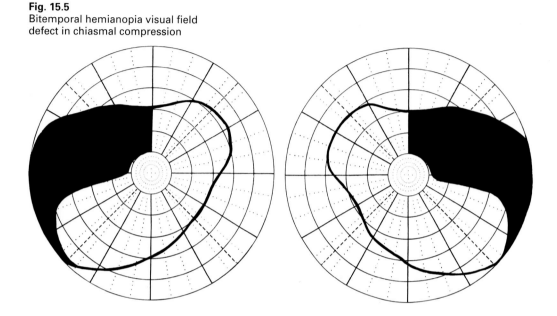

Other lesions which can cause similar bitemporal hemianopia are craniopharyngioma (mainly in children), suprasellar meningioma and carotid aneurysms although these aneurysms give rise to more rapid symptoms.

Investigations consist of computed tomography (CT) scan, carotid arteriography and full endocrine assessment.

Most expanding chromophobe adenomata pituitary tumours require surgical removal. The eosinophil adenomata giving rise to the clinical picture of *acromegaly* and *gigantism* frequently spare the optic chiasma and their removal is not often required.

OPTIC TRACT, OPTIC RADIATION AND VISUAL CORTEX CONDITIONS

Vascular
Occlusion of branches of the middle cerebral and posterior cerebral arteries cause sudden loss of vision in one half of the visual field in each eye (homonymous hemianopia).

Conditions causing this are hypertension, diabetes mellitus, cranial arteritis, blood dyscrasias and emboli from the heart, internal carotid and vertebral arteries.

Cerebral tumours
An expanding primary or secondary tumour may compress the visual pathway behind the chiasma giving rise to a homonymous hemianopia.

Multiple sclerosis and meningitis
Homonymous hemianopia may occur in these diseases.

The symptoms and signs
In vascular lesions behind the optic chiasma the patient notices sudden loss of vision in one half of the visual field in each eye. He commonly only notices the visual field loss in the eye with the larger temporal field loss and fails to notice the similar loss in the nasal field of the other eye. This visual field loss is gradual in onset with cerebral tumours.

Examination shows normal pupil light reflexes, normal fundi and a homonymous hemianopia on one side, right or left (Fig. 15.6).

Fig. 15.6
Homonymous hemianopia visual field defect

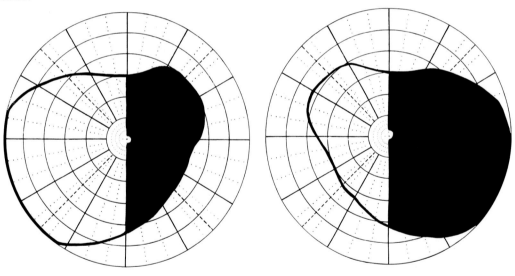

SUMMARY OF VISUAL FIELD DEFECTS OF THE VISUAL PATHWAYS

Retina Optic nerve	Visual field defect on side of affected eye only
Chiasma	Bitemporal (heteronymous) hemianopia (Fig. 15.5)
Optic tract Optic radiations Visual cortex	Homonymous hemianopia (Fig. 15.6)

Index

134